Lung Cancer Screening

Editor

GAETANO ROCCO

THORACIC
SURGERY CLINICS

www.thoracic.theclinics.com

Consulting Editor
M. BLAIR MARSHALL

May 2015 • Volume 25 • Number 2

ELSEVIER

1600 John F. Kennedy Boulevard • Suite 1800 • Philadelphia, Pennsylvania, 19103-2899

http://www.thoracic.theclinics.com

THORACIC SURGERY CLINICS Volume 25, Number 2
May 2015 ISSN 1547-4127, ISBN-13: 978-0-323-37621-1

Editor: John Vassallo (j.vassallo@elsevier.com)
Developmental Editor: Stephanie Carter

Thoracic Surgery Clinics (ISSN 1547-4127) is published quarterly by Elsevier Inc., 360 Park Avenue South, New York, NY 10010-1710. Months of publication are February, May, August, and November. Business and editorial offices: 1600 John F. Kennedy Boulevard, Suite 1800, Philadelphia, PA 19103-2899. Periodicals postage paid at New York, NY, and additional mailing offices. Subscription prices are $350.00 per year (US individuals), $453.00 per year (US institutions), $165.00 per year (US Students), $435.00 per year (Canadian individuals), $585.00 per year (Canadian institutions), $225.00 per year (Canadian and international students), $465.00 per year (international individuals), and $585.00 per year (international institutions). Foreign air speed delivery is included in all Clinics' subscription prices. All prices are subject to change without notice. **POSTMASTER:** Send address changes to Thoracic Surgery Clinics, Elsevier Health Sciences Division, Subscription Customer Service, 3251 Riverport Lane, Maryland Heights, MO 63043. **Customer Service (orders, claims, online, change of address): Telephone: 1-800-654-2452 (U.S. and Canada); 314-447-8871 (outside U.S. and Canada). Fax: 314-447-8029. E-mail: journalscustomerservice-usa@elsevier.com (for print support); journalsonlinesupport-usa@elsevier.com (for online support).**

Reprints. For copies of 100 or more, of articles in this publication, please contact Commercial Rights Department, Elsevier Inc., 360 Park Avenue South, New York, NY 10010-1710. Tel: 212-633-3874; Fax: 212-633-3820; E-mail: reprints@elsevier.com.

Thoracic Surgery Clinics is covered in *MEDLINE/PubMed (Index Medicus), EMBASE/Excerpta Medica, Science Citation Index Expanded (SciSearch®), Journal Citation Reports/Science Edition,* and *Current Contents®/Clinical Medicine.*

Contributors

CONSULTING EDITOR

M. BLAIR MARSHALL, MD, FACS
Chief, Division of Thoracic Surgery; Associate
Professor of Surgery, Department of Surgery,
Georgetown University Medical Center,
Georgetown University School of Medicine,
Washington, DC

EDITOR

**GAETANO ROCCO, MD, FRCS(Ed),
FETCS, FCCP**
Chief, Division of Thoracic Surgery;
Director, Department of Thoracic Surgery
and Oncology, Istituto Nazionale Tumori,
Fondazione Pascale, IRCCS, Naples, Italy

AUTHORS

PRASAD S. ADUSUMILLI, MD
Associate Attending, Thoracic Service,
Department of Surgery, Memorial Sloan
Kettering Cancer Center, New York,
New York

MARK S. ALLEN, MD
Professor of Surgery, Mayo Clinic, Rochester,
Minnesota

NASSER ALTORKI, MD
Professor of Cardiothoracic Surgery,
Weill Cornell Medical College, New York,
New York

SHANDA H. BLACKMON, MD, MPH, FACS
Associate Professor, Thoracic Surgery, Mayo
Clinic, Rochester, Minnesota

PAOLO BOFFETTA, MD, MPH
Professor of Hematology and Oncology,
Icahn School of Medicine at Mount Sinai,
New York, New York

PETER R. BUCCIARELLI, MD
Research Fellow, Thoracic Service,
Department of Surgery, Memorial Sloan
Kettering Cancer Center, New York,
New York

NEEL P. CHUDGAR, MD
Research Fellow, Thoracic Service,
Department of Surgery, Memorial Sloan
Kettering Cancer Center, New York,
New York

JANET P. EDWARDS, MD, MPH, FRCSC
Thoracic Surgery Resident, Department of
Surgery, Foothills Medical Centre, University of
Calgary, Calgary, Alberta, Canada

SHAMIRAM R. FEINGLASS, MD, MPH
CEO, The Feinglass Group, Warsaw,
Indiana

ERIN A. GILLASPIE, MD
Mayo Clinic, Rochester, Minnesota

SEAN C. GRONDIN, MD, MPH, FRCSC, FACS
Clinical Associate Professor of Surgery, Department of Surgery, Foothills Medical Centre, University of Calgary, Calgary, Alberta, Canada

CLAUDIA I. HENSCHKE, PhD, MD
Professor of Radiology, Icahn School of Medicine at Mount Sinai, New York, New York

ELIZABETH M. JEFFRIES
Research Assistant, Thoracic Service, Department of Surgery, Memorial Sloan Kettering Cancer Center, New York, New York

DAVID R. JONES, MD
Professor and Chief, Thoracic Service, Department of Surgery, Memorial Sloan Kettering Cancer Center, New York, New York

SETH B. KRANTZ, MD
Fellow, Division of Cardiothoracic Surgery, Department of Surgery, Washington University School of Medicine, St Louis, Missouri

DAVID C. MAUCHLEY, MD
Chief Resident, Division of Cardiothoracic Surgery, University of Colorado School of Medicine, Aurora, Colorado

BRYAN F. MEYERS, MD
Patrick and Joy Williamson Professor of Surgery; Chief, Section of Thoracic Surgery, Division of Cardiothoracic Surgery, Department of Surgery, Washington University School of Medicine, St Louis, Missouri

JOHN D. MITCHELL, MD
Professor and Chief, Section of General Thoracic Surgery, Division of Cardiothoracic Surgery, University of Colorado School of Medicine, Aurora, Colorado

BERNARD J. PARK, MD
Deputy Chief of Clinical Affairs, Thoracic Service, Department of Surgery, Memorial Sloan Kettering Cancer Center, New York, New York

UGO PASTORINO, MD
Division of Thoracic Surgery, Fondazione IRCCS Istituto Nazionale dei Tumori, Milan, Italy

JESPER HOLST PEDERSEN, MD, DMSc
Chief Surgeon; Associate Professor, Department of Cardiothoracic Surgery, Rigshospitalet, University of Copenhagen, Copenhagen, Denmark

NABIL P. RIZK, MD
Associate Attending, Thoracic Service, Department of Surgery, Memorial Sloan Kettering Cancer Center, New York, New York

GAETANO ROCCO, MD, FRCS(Ed), FETCS, FCCP
Chief, Division of Thoracic Surgery; Director, Department of Thoracic Surgery and Oncology, Istituto Nazionale Tumori, Fondazione Pascale, IRCCS, Naples, Italy

JENS BENN SØRENSEN, MD, DMSc, MPA
Associate Professor; Chief Physician, Department of Oncology, Finsen Centre, Rigshospitalet, University of Copenhagen, Copenhagen, Denmark

MARIO SILVA, MD
Division of Thoracic Surgery, Fondazione IRCCS Istituto Nazionale dei Tumori, Milan; Section of Radiology, Department of Surgical Sciences, University of Parma, Parma, Italy

GIULIA VERONESI, MD
Thoracic Surgeon; Director, Lung Cancer Early Detection Unit, European Institute of Oncology, Milan, Italy

DOUGLAS E. WOOD, MD, FACS
Professor and Chief, Division of Cardiothoracic Surgery; Vice-Chair, Department of Surgery, Endowed Chair in Lung Cancer Research, University of Washington, Seattle, Washington

DAVID F. YANKELEVITZ, MD
Professor of Radiology, Icahn School of Medicine at Mount Sinai, New York, New York

Contents

The Mayo Clinic has been involved in screening for lung cancer since the lung cancer project in 1971. The Mayo Clinic recently completed a study of more than 1500 patients with low-dose computed tomographic (CT) screening for lung cancer. Results showed that more than 75% of patients in the screening program had a lung nodule but only a small percentage had lung cancer. As others have found, screening with low-dose CT finds patients with lung cancer at an earlier stage and hopefully will increase the cure rate.

The International Early Lung Cancer Action Program (I-ELCAP) used a novel study design that provided quantitative information about annual CT screening for lung cancer. The results stimulated additional studies of lung cancer screening and ultimately led to the National Lung Screening Trial (NLST) being initiated in 2002, as the initial report in 1999 was sufficiently compelling to reawaken interest in screening for lung cancer. The authors think that the I-ELCAP and NLST "story" provides a strong argument for relevant agencies to consider alternative study designs for the public funding of studies aimed at evaluating the effectiveness of screening and other medical trials.

The National Lung Screening Trial was a large, multicenter, randomized controlled trial published in 2011. It found that annual screening with low-dose CT (LDCT) in a high-risk population was associated with a 20% reduction in lung cancer–specific mortality compared with conventional chest radiography. Several leading professional organizations have since put forth lung cancer screening guidelines that include the use of LDCT, largely on the basis of this study. Broad adoption of these screening recommendations, however, remains a challenge.

Results of the recent National Lung Cancer Screening Trial show a significant survival benefit for annual screening with a low-dose computed tomographic (CT) scan in high-risk individuals. This result has led the US Preventive Services Task Force to recommend annual low-dose CT scans for this at-risk population. Less well characterized are the risks from screening. The primary risks from screening are radiation exposure, false-positive results and unnecessary diagnostic and therapeutic procedures, overdiagnosis and overtreatment, and increased psychological distress. This article reviews these risks, which must be considered and weighed against the benefits when discussing enrollment with patients.

European studies have contributed significantly to the understanding of lung cancer screening. Smoking within screening, quality of life, nodule management, minimally invasive treatments, cancer prevention programs, and risk models have been extensively investigated by European groups. Mortality data from European screening studies have not been encouraging so far, but long-term results of the NELSON study are eagerly awaited. Investigations on molecular markers of lung cancer are ongoing in Europe; preliminary results suggest they may become an important screening tool in the future.

To understand the challenges of screening for lung cancer, surgeons should be familiar with fundamental epidemiologic concepts pertaining to screening and have an understanding of the evidence regarding the various modalities used for screening lung cancer. One large, recent study has confirmed that screening for lung cancer with low-dose computed tomography decreases mortality in high-risk individuals. As a result of these findings, comprehensive screening programs are being developed. High-quality programs should be safe, cost-effective, accessible to high-risk patients, and involve the participation of a multidisciplinary team. Surgeons should be engaged in the implementation of screening programs for lung cancer.

The National Comprehensive Cancer Network (NCCN), a not-for-profit alliance of 25 of the world's leading cancer centers devoted to patient care, research, and education, is dedicated to improving the quality, effectiveness, and efficiency of cancer care so that patients can live better lives. The intent of the NCCN Guidelines is to assist in the decision-making process of individuals involved in cancer care—including physicians, nurses, pharmacists, payers, patients, and their families—with the ultimate goal of advancing patient care in the fight against cancer.

In 2013, the United States Preventive Services Task Force made a grade B recommendation for annual screening for lung cancer with low-dose computed tomography in adult patients 55 to 80 years of age who have a 30 pack-year smoking history and currently smoke or have quit within the last 15 years. In practical terms, the

United States Preventive Services Task Force recommendations will likely mean a large increase in actual screening rates.

The United States Preventive Services Task Force recently endorsed the use of low-dose computed tomography for lung cancer screening in high-risk patients because of the potential to reduce deaths. Before implementation on a national level, it will be important to ensure that a safe, high-quality, and accessible service can be adequately provided. It will also be important to make sure that screening is cost-effective. This article summarizes the published analyses of lung cancer screening cost, provides a contemporary estimation of the annual cost of screening in the United States, and identifies areas for improvement in the future.

The selection of populations to be screened for lung cancer must be further optimized before translation to large population. A 3-step refinement should be integrated into forthcoming lung cancer trials, namely, calculation of risk based on (1) demographics, (2) biological factors, and (3) radiologic inputs. Biological sampling should be implemented up-front to reduce the use of low-dose computed tomography scanning in patients with lower risk of aggressive disease and, notably, to improve detection of aggressive disease that is overlooked by current screening strategies.

Benefits and risks of computed tomography lung cancer screening are discussed with specific focus on oncologic and financial issues. Earlier disease stage at diagnosis implies that more patients are treated surgically, but the changes in oncologic treatment will not be dramatic. The crucial issue for implementation of screening will be that it is cost effective. Preliminary data from the National Lung Screening Trial indicate that it is cost effective and comparable to screening for other major malignancies. Some future modifications in the computed tomography screening methodology are discussed.

THORACIC SURGERY CLINICS

Preface
Lung Cancer Screening

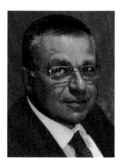

Gaetano Rocco, MD, FRCS(Ed), FETCS, FCCP
Editor

Until the National Lung Screening Trial (NLST), the results of lung cancer screening had been considered controversial if not useless in the fight against the most ominous among the common cancers. It seemed like we had to resign ourselves to the idea that smoking cessation would be the only effective preventative measure. The results from NLST have brought about new hope by producing a 20% reduction of lung cancer mortality, albeit at the same time raising several legitimate questions on its indiscriminate implementation on a wider national scale. This issue of *Thoracic Surgery Clinics* devoted to lung cancer screening is meant to guide the reader through a detailed analysis of past screening models (Mayo and ELCAP) to understand the impact of NLST, along with the ongoing European studies, on health policies and costs in both the United States and Europe. Furthermore, the modality for surgeon involvement in lung cancer screening programs is discussed with a closer focus on the need for wider adoption of minimally invasive techniques and of

(biomolecular) strategies aimed at the reduction of false positives to minimize the resort to unnecessary surgery. Finally, the outlook on the long-term perspectives of lung cancer screening is analyzed to ascertain whether the glimmer of hope generated with the NLST will be shining brighter in the future. In fact, the evidence in favor of lung cancer screening is piling up to the point that, shortly after this issue was completed, the Centers for Medicare and Medicaid Services in the United States proposed adding screening for lung cancer with low-dose computed tomography, once per year for appropriate candidates.

Gaetano Rocco, MD, FRCS(Ed), FETCS, FCCP
Istituto Nazionale Tumori
Fondazione Pascale, IRCCS
Via Mariano Semmola 81
Naples 80131, Italy

E-mail address:
gaetano.rocco@btopenworld.com

Thorac Surg Clin 25 (2015) ix
http://dx.doi.org/10.1016/j.thorsurg.2014.12.006
1547-4127/15/$ – see front matter © 2015 Published by Elsevier Inc.

thoracic.theclinics.com

Computed Tomographic Screening for Lung Cancer: The Mayo Clinic Experience

Erin A. Gillaspie, MD, Mark S. Allen, MD*

KEYWORDS

- Lung cancer • Screening • Low-dose CT • Prevention

KEY POINTS

- Screening with low-dose computed tomography (LDCT) reduces lung cancer mortality.
- Results from screening for lung cancer need to be carefully managed to avoid unnecessary surgery.
- Screening using LDCT is superior to screening with chest roentgenograms.

BACKGROUND

Lung cancer has long stood as the most lethal cancer faced by the medical profession. An estimated 1.6 million patients worldwide are expected to die this year of lung cancer, which accounts for 19% of all cancer deaths.[1]

The most important risk factor for the development of lung cancer remains smoking. Despite the plethora of evidence proving the detriments of smoking, approximately 18% of the adult US population continues to smoke.[2] The relative risk of developing lung cancer is 25 times higher in a smoker than in a nonsmoker.[3] Still, there are other risks to consider including family history, chronic obstructive pulmonary disease, idiopathic pulmonary fibrosis, environmental radon exposure, passive smoking, asbestos exposure, and certain occupational exposures.

Lung cancer presentation varies from indolent and subtle symptoms to persistent cough, hemoptysis, chest pain, or recurrent pneumonia or bronchitis. Too often, the presentation of lung cancer with symptoms leads to the finding of an advanced-stage cancer that is unlikely to be cured.

Screening examinations for lung cancer have significantly lagged behind those for other types of cancers including colon, breast, and prostate cancer, all of which have a significantly better survival.

BENEFITS OF EARLY DETECTION

The stage at presentation determines the overall survival. Approximately 46% of patients with lung cancer present at an advanced stage with limited treatment options.[4] A screening tool that could provide an earlier diagnosis would potentially shift a significant number of patients into a stage with more treatment options.

For the past 5 decades, the Mayo Clinic has participated in efforts to establish a protocol for the earlier detection of lung cancer.

CHEST RADIOGRAPH AS A SCREENING TOOL: THE MAYO LUNG PROJECT
Study Design

The Mayo Lung Project (MLP) was a randomized controlled study conducted between 1971 and 1983. The study accrued 10,933 male outpatients who were known smokers and not suspected of having lung cancer. These patients underwent a baseline screening with chest radiograph (CXR)

Disclosures: the authors have nothing to disclose.
Mayo Clinic, Rochester, MN 55905, USA
* Corresponding author. Department of Surgery, 200 First Street, SouthWest, Rochester, MN 55905.
E-mail address: Allen.mark@mayo.edu

Thorac Surg Clin 25 (2015) 121–127
http://dx.doi.org/10.1016/j.thorsurg.2014.11.001
1547-4127/15/$ – see front matter © 2015 Elsevier Inc. All rights reserved.

and sputum cytology (prevalence study). Patients with a negative result of CXR and a life expectancy of greater than 5 years were invited to participate in a randomized controlled trial of lung cancer incidence. Ultimately, 9211 men were randomly assigned to receive either the standard of care at Mayo for the 1970's, which was annual CXR and sputum cytology, or to belong to the intervention arm in which participants underwent CXR and sputum cytology every 4 months for 6 years (incidence studies). There was 75% compliance in the intervention arm of the study. Follow-up of the MLP concluded in 1983.[5]

Results from the Study

The prevalence CXRs revealed 91 previously undiagnosed lung carcinomas (8.3 per 1000 screened). Of these, half were early-stage cancers and were amenable to resection. Overall, the 5-year survival for these patients was 40%.

Over the next 6 years, an additional 206 (5.5 per 1000 person-years) cases of lung carcinoma were diagnosed in the intervention arm compared with 160 (4.3 per 1000 person-years) in the control group. The additional cases diagnosed in the intervention arm were early-stage cancers.[6]

Mortality

The incidence of lung cancer and the stage at which it was diagnosed differed between the 2 arms of the study. The median survival for patients who were diagnosed with lung cancer in the intervention arm was 1.3 years versus 0.9 years in the usual care arm.

For resected, early-stage disease (T1 or T2 lesions), the median survival was 16 years for the intervention arm compared with only 5 years in the usual care arm. Treatment was the same in each group, with 81% and 80% of patients in the intervention and usual care groups, respectively, going on to have resection. In advanced-stage lung cancer, survival rates were same in both arms of the study.

Despite these differences in survival, the values never reached statistical significant ($P = .16$). Therefore, it was concluded that more frequent examinations with CXR and sputum cytology did not seem to confer a survival benefit and therefore these should not be used as screening tools.[6]

Extended Follow-up for the Mayo Lung Project

In 1996, the National Death Index (NDI) was used to provide extended follow-up on any remaining MLP patients who were still alive at the conclusion of the study in 1983. Medical records and the NDI database were reviewed for clinical status, and if deceased, the date and cause.

Of the 6523 patients remaining at the end of the study, 2961 patients had available data for review. After 13 years, death totals for the study were 303 patients in the usual care arm and 337 in the intervention arm. The median follow-up was 20 years. Lung cancer mortality rate was calculated to be 4.4 per 1000 person-years in the intervention arm and 3.9 deaths per 1000 person-years in the usual care arm. There was no statistical difference. All-cause mortality also did not differ by study arm.

The data were adjusted for lung cancer risk modifiers including age, smoking, exposure to nontobacco lung carcinogens, and history of pulmonary illnesses, and the mortality rates did not differ significantly between the 2 study arms.[7]

Case Survival

No reduction in lung cancer mortality was seen in the intervention arm of the MLP. However, a case survival difference was observed at 1, 5, 10, and 15 years. One year after the diagnosis of lung cancer, survival was 61.7% for patients participating in the intervention arm compared with 50.1% in the usual care arm. Similar trends were seen in continued follow-up at 5, 10, and 15 years.

The extended follow-up and reevaluation of data still could not conclude that CXR was an appropriate modality for screening for lung cancer despite trends to improved survival.[7]

Comparable Trials

Similar studies were conducted to evaluate the effectiveness of CXR in screening for lung cancer. The Prostate, Lung, Colorectal and Ovarian (PLCO) randomized trial, for example, offered annual CXR to patients for 4 years versus no screening. Groups were well matched. Annual screening with CXR did not reduce lung cancer mortality compared with usual care.[8]

Computed Tomographic Scan as a Screening Tool

The computed tomographic (CT) scan was first used clinically in the 1970s. During that time, scans required high radiation dosages and long image acquisition times. These requirements made CT an impractical modality for screening.

As CT scanning technology improved with superior image quality, thinner slices, and faster acquisition of imaging, many groups began to study the CT scan as a screening tool for lung cancer. Detractors of CT screening cited radiation exposure as a prohibitive risk. The cumulative dose of radiation for a screening test was deemed inappropriate if the screening test could ultimately result in pathologic condition including cancer.

In 1990, studies began to emerge suggesting that image quality for diagnostic purposes could be maintained at lower milliamperage settings.

The Mayo Clinic, among other institutions, worked to demonstrate the utility of LDCT scanning as a screening tool.

Minimal Tube Current Maintains Image Quality

The development of LDCT greatly reduced the radiation doses that patients were exposed to and the scan times, making increased usage of CT as a scanning tool reasonable.

Dr Mayo of Vancouver Hospital and Dr Hartman of Mayo Clinic at the respective departments of radiology studied the minimal tube current required to obtain adequate image quality to detect lung and mediastinal abnormalities in CT scanning.

A total of 30 patients undergoing standard CT scan of the chest (at 400 mA) had 4 additional sections imaged at reduced current (200, 140, 80, and 20 mA) performed at 2 different levels. CT scans were reviewed by 2 radiologists who were blinded to the CT scan technique. Image quality was maintained at 200 and 140 mA but was noted to be significantly inferior at lower levels. However, there was no significant difference in the rate of detection of mediastinal or lung parenchymal abnormalities between any of the imaging techniques.

The study concluded that a reduced current of 140 mA could be used with preserved image quality and equivalent rate of detection of abnormalities.[9] **Fig. 1** demonstrates imaging obtained through routine chest CT protocol and through reduced current level.

IMPLEMENTING A COMPUTED TOMOGRAPHIC SCREENING PROTOCOL FOR LUNG CANCER
Mayo Clinic Screening Protocol

The Mayo Clinic CT screening study began in January 1999 and continued through December 2002. The study enrolled 1520 participants who met the following criteria: age greater than 50, current or former smokers of more than 20 pack years, and having quit less than 10 years ago.

Each patient underwent a baseline (prevalence) chest CT, followed by 3 subsequent annual (incidence) CT scans. Scans were performed at low-level doses and reviewed by 1 of 4 chest radiologists. In addition, sputum samples were obtained annually, as well as blood samples, which were stored for subsequent DNA analysis.

Nodule management recommendations were created internally at Mayo and shared with referring physicians. Follow-up was determined at their discretion. For nodules smaller than 4 mm, repeat CT scan at 6 months was recommended; for nodules 4 to 8 mm, a repeat scan in 3 months was recommended; for nodules 8 to 20 mm, a thin-slice CT scan was recommended with consideration for positron emission tomography (PET); and nodules greater than 20 mm were recommended for biopsy. Nodules that remained stable in size for over 2 years were defined as benign.

Follow-up after baseline imaging was excellent with 98% participation. After 3 years of screening, 2832 uncalcified pulmonary nodules were identified. Ultimately, 40 primary lung cancers were diagnosed. Of these, 26 were identified with the prevalence CT scan, 10 were diagnosed at incidence CT scan, 2 were interval cancers, and 2 were diagnosed by sputum cytology alone.

Pulmonary resections were performed in 31 of 40 participants, and 21 (60%) of 40 patients were at stage IA at diagnosis.

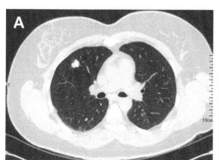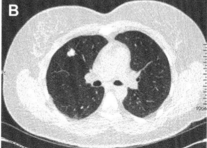

Fig. 1. (A) Image acquired with routine chest CT protocol. (B) Simulated image at a dose level that is a quarter of the routine dose. (From Yu L, Shiung M, Jondal D, et al. Development and validation of practical lower-dose-simulation tool for optimizing computed tomography scan protocols. J Comput Assist Tomogr 2012;36(4):477–88; with permission.)

In addition to the 40 lung cancers diagnosed by CT screening, there were 696 clinically significant findings. Also, interestingly by the conclusion of the study, 79% of patients participating had at least 1 pulmonary nodule.

Most lung cancers diagnosed in this study were stage IA. Certainly, the high rate of stage I portents superior survival for asymptomatic patients diagnosed by CT scan: 62% to 82% at 5 years. It was concluded that LDCT scan served as a good screening modality for high-risk patients.

Unfortunately, it is not clear from the study whether these findings are simply because of screening or are affected by confounding factors including selection bias, overdiagnosis, and lead time bias.[10]

Other studies including the National Lung Cancer Screening Trial (NLST) also show survival benefit with CT screening, lending some credence to the above-mentioned findings.

The Surgical Considerations

Mayo Clinic enrolled 1112 patients from January 1999 to December 2002 in a lung cancer screening study with the hypothesis that CT scan in the appropriate population of patients would lead to improved detection at earlier stages and improved treatment with survival. In the 1112 patients in the study, there were 3130 indeterminate pulmonary nodules; 51 patients underwent 60 thoracic operations for a variety of indications (**Fig. 2**).

The number of nodules identified at the time of surgery ranged from 1 to 7 with a median of 3. Nodules were monitored for a median of 4.3 months before surgical intervention. Further examinations were performed in several patients: thin-section CT scan in 25 patients, PET scan in 16 patients, bronchoscopy in 5 patients, and transthoracic needle aspiration in 5 cases.

Type of operation performed included lobectomy in 37 patients, wedge resection in 11, segmentectomy in 6, video assisted thoracic surgery (VATS) pleurodesis in 1, bilobectomy in 2, mediastinoscopy in 2, and anterior mediastinotomy in 1 patient. Overall, 79 nodules were resected. Benign disease was found in 18.1% of cases. Lung cancer was found in 81.9% (45 cases). Cell types for the cancers were predominantly adenocarcinoma (15), followed by adenocarcinoma in situ (13 patients), squamous cell carcinoma (15), carcinoid (2), small cell cancer (2), and large cell cancer (1). Stage at the time of diagnosis is represented in **Fig. 3**.

Postoperative complications occurred in 27% patients. These included prolonged air leak, atrial arrhythmias, pneumonia, ileus, cerebral vascular accident (CVS), depression, and vocal cord paralysis. There was also 1 operative mortality secondary to intracerebral hemorrhage.

CT finds a large number of indeterminate pulmonary nodules in smokers aged 50 years or older most of which are observed and not operated on. The malignancies identified represent only 1.5% of the nodules identified.

Management of indeterminate nodules poses a significant diagnostic and therapeutic challenge. Screening high-risk population with LDCT results in the detection of numerous pulmonary nodules, most of which are benign.

The small diameter of most of the pulmonary nodules limits the usefulness of some of the diagnostic imaging modalities. PET and CT of the chest are limited to nodules that are 1 cm or more in diameter. This size limitation actually excludes 25% of all nodules and 16% of the malignant nodules. Invasive diagnostic procedures are also limited by size and anatomic location.

Mortality associated with surgical resection was low at 1.7%. Fortunately, no deaths

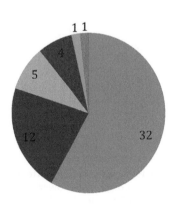

■ Enlarging nodule

■ New nodule

■ Positive CT nodule enhancement

■ Worrisome morphologic appearance

■ Enlarging mediastinal nodes

■ Represents spontaneous pneumothorax

Fig. 2. Indication for surgery in 55 patients undergoing procedures for concerning-appearing nodules on CT scan.

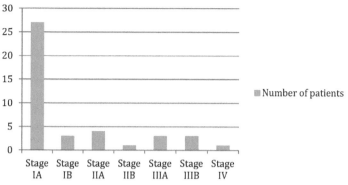

Fig. 3. Surgical staging of lung cancer.

occurred among the patients found to have only benign disease. Morbidity was significant, indicating that pulmonary resections should not be undertaken lightly. Careful patient selection is critical.[11]

SHORTCOMINGS OF THE COMPUTED TOMOGRAPHIC SCREENING
Patient Factors

There are many factors that have been shown to increase the incidence of lung cancer in addition to smoking. Many studies, including the NLST, do not account for race, body mass index, the presence of chronic obstructive pulmonary disease (COPD) or emphysema, or personal and family history. All these factors have been shown to be independent predictors of lung cancer.[12]

The Mayo Clinic reviewed patients diagnosed with lung cancer. Of 14,370 patients seen over a 4-year period (2007–2011), only 33.6% fit the NLST criteria for screening. Therefore 66% of patients who developed lung cancer would not have been eligible for screening based on the requirements (Yang, unpublished data, 2012). The creation of a risk score could help to obviate some of these shortcomings.

Most patients who are left out in the NLST would be former smokers (often having quit more than 15 years prior) but remaining at high risk. The number needed to be screened would be 3 times that suggested in the NLST (1 life saved for 320 people screened) to pick up additional cases.[13]

The National Comprehensive Cancer Network was the first organization to create guidelines for LDCT screening for lung cancer.[14] The American College of Chest Physicians and the American Society of Clinical Oncology have both released statements supporting screening that meet NLST guidelines.[15,16] The American Association of Thoracic Surgery also recommends annual screening for those who meet the NLST criteria, but they include patients who are aged 50 years and older, have a 20-year smoking history, or have any additional cumulative risk of developing lung cancer that is 5% or greater over the ensuing 5 years.[17]

Cost of Screening

The cost of lung cancer screening is significant. Data were collected from the 2009 National Health Interview Survey by the Center for Medicaid and Medicare Services and the NLST. Then an economic model to predict the cost per life saved by lung cancer screening was created. The cost of LDCT screening in the United States could range from $1.3 to $2.0 billion dollars in annual health care expenditure. Of the patients who are screened, approximately 8100 premature lung cancer deaths would be prevented. The calculated cost of screening to avoid 1 cancer death is approximately $240,000.[18] Other studies have estimated life saved to cost anywhere from $19,000 to the $169,000.[19,20]

Length of Screening

The frequency and total duration of screening has yet to be completely defined. Many experts would advocate that eligibility for screening be calculated for each individual patient. Patients should continue to undergo annual screening until their risk of cancer falls below a set threshold (because of length of smoking cessation) or until debility.

Overdiagnosis and False Positives

Only 1.3% of patients in the Mayo study had pulmonary nodules that were proven to be cancer, which leaves 99% of pulmonary nodules representing false-positive findings.[11] Assuming that most patients will have at least one positive CT examination after a few years of CT screening, despite excellent health care teams managing these patients, many patients will undergo additional studies for benign findings. The PLuSS (Pittsburgh Lung Screening Study) and ITALUNG (Italian Lung Project) trials demonstrated an 18% to 34% rate of surgical procedures for benign histology.[21,22] The NELSON (Dutch-Belgian Randomized Lung Cancer Screening Trial [Dutch Acronym: NELSON]) trial confirmed that 27% of surgeries performed were for benign disease.[23] There are financial and emotional costs associated with overdiagnosis, along with the potential morbidity and mortality of surgical intervention.

A large proportion of cancers diagnosed were stage IA. These may represent a subset of cancer with a more indolent growth pattern and could be clinically insignificant. Could these be lesions that patients will die with and not of?[24] There will be several nonpulmonary findings that will also necessitate follow-up and treatment.

The Difficulties of Implementation

The implementation of a nationwide or even worldwide CT screening protocol poses challenges. Published studies, including the NLST, Mayo, NELSON, and so forth, were carried out in a center of excellence with experienced radiologists, pulmonologists, thoracic surgeons, and medical and radiation oncologists. Can similar results be replicated in small institutions that do not boast this robust subspecialty support?

Continued Smoking

Screening is costly, and so is treatment. It would be appropriate to mandate smoking cessation in patients who would like to participate in lung cancer screening. Unfortunately, the structure of the eligibility criteria included in present screening recommendations unintentionally endorses continued smoking. For patients who quit smoking at the age of 55, in 15 years they will no longer meet the criteria to continue screening despite having a higher risk at the age of 70 of having lung cancer. In this way, the NLST screening protocols promote continued smoking.

SUMMARY

There is still much that remains to be determined with lung cancer screening. There are many challenges to overcome. First is the lack of consensus on who to screen. Major thoracic organizations all have differing recommendations as to the appropriate population to include. At present at Mayo, a modification to the NLST guidelines has been implemented. The Tammemagi calculator is used to identify patients at high risk of lung cancer,

and these patients are entered into the screening protocol.

Also concerning is that no study has demonstrated that screening can be carried out successfully outside of major academic centers. Furthermore, it is still unknown whether Medicare will reimburse for the study, which would significantly reduce the population eligible for screening.

Technology continues to improve, and many efforts at Mayo have been focused on reducing the radiation dose in lung cancer CT screening. Iterative reconstruction has been used to improve the image quality, which can be translated into a substantial dose reduction. More recently, X-ray spectrum optimization has improved the dose efficiency in CT scanning, which has allowed the dose of a screening CT to be reduced to the level that is close to that of a few CXRs. These advances will allow CT scanning to function as an excellent screening tool for lung cancer and allow us to reduce the mortality from lung cancer.

REFERENCES

1. Ferlay J, Soerjomataram I, Ervik M. Cancer incidence and mortality worldwide: IARC cancer base no. 11. GLOBOCAN, International Agency for Research on Cancer. 2013. Available at: http://globocan.iarc.fr.
2. Centers for Disease Control and Prevention. Current cigarette smoking among adults—United States, 2005–2012. MMWR Morb Mortal Wkly Rep 2014; 63(02):29–34.
3. U.S. Department of Health and Human Services. The health consequences of smoking-50 years of progress: a report of the surgeon general. Atlanta (GA): United States Government; 2014.
4. Detterbeck FC, Boffa DJ, Tanoue LT, et al. The new lung cancer staging system. Chest 2009;136(1): 260–71.
5. Fontana RS, Sanderson DR, Woolner LB, et al. The Mayo Lung Project for early detection and localization of bronchogenic carcinoma: a status report. Chest 1975;61:511–22.
6. Fontana RS, Sanderson DR, Taylor WF, et al. Early lung cancer detection: results of the initial (prevalence) radiologic and cytologic screening in the Mayo Clinic Study. Am Rev Respir Dis 1984;130:561–5.
7. Marcus PM, Bergstralh EJ, Fagerstrom RM, et al. Lung cancer mortality in the mayo lung project: impact of the extended follow-up. J Natl Cancer Inst 2000;92(16):1308–16.
8. Oken MM, Hocking WG, Kvale PA, et al. Screening by chest radiograph and lung cancer mortality: the Prostate, Lung, Colorectal and Ovarian (PLCO) randomized trial. JAMA 2011;306(17):1865–73.
9. Mayo JR, Hartman TE, Lee KS, et al. CT of the chest: minimal tube current required for good image quality

with the least radiation dose. AJR Am J Roentgenol 1995;164:603–7.

10. Swensen SJ, Jett JR, Hartman TE, et al. Lung cancer screening with CT: Mayo Clinic Experience. Radiology 2003;226:756–61.

11. Crestanello JA, Allen MS, Jett JR, et al. Thoracic surgical operations in patients enrolled in a computed tomographic screening trial. J Thorac Cardiovasc Surg 2004;128:254–9.

12. Tammemagi MC, Katki HA, Hocking WG, et al. Selection criteria for lung-cancer screening. N Engl J Med 2013;368:728–36.

13. Aberle DR, Adams AM, Berg CD, et al. Reduced lung-cancer mortality with low-dose computed tomographic screening. N Engl J Med 2011;365:395–409.

14. NCCN guidelines. Available at: www.nccn.org.

15. Editorial Board. Expert perspective from ASCO on the results of the National Lung Cancer Screening Trial. Cancer.net Articles. 2012.

16. Detterbeck FC, Mazzone PJ, Naidich DP, et al. Screening for lung cancer: diagnosis and management of lung cancer, 3rd ed. American College of Chest Physicians evidence-based clinical practice guidelines. Chest 2013;143:e78S.

17. Jaklitsch MT, Jacobson FL, Austin JH, et al. The American Association for Thoracic Surgery guidelines for lung cancer screening using low-dose computed tomography scans for lung cancer

survivors and other high-risk groups. J Thorac Cardiovasc Surg 2012;144(1):33–8.

18. Goulart BH, Bensink ME, Mummy DG, et al. Lung cancer screening with low-dose computed tomography: costs, national expenditures, and cost-effectiveness. J Natl Compr Canc Netw 2012;10(2):267–75.

19. McMahon PM, Kong CY, Bouzan C, et al. Cost-effectiveness of computed tomography screening for lung cancer in the United States. J Thorac Oncol 2011;6:1841–8.

20. Pyenson BS, Sander MS, Jiang Y, et al. An actuarial analysis shows that offering lung cancer screening as an insurance benefit would save lives at relatively low cost. Health Aff 2012;31:771–9.

21. Wilson DO, Weissfeld JL, Fuhrman CR, et al. The Pittsburgh lung screening study (PLuSS)L Outcomes within 3 years of a first computed tomography scan. Am J Respir Crit Care Med 2008;127:956–61.

22. Lopes Pegna A, Picozzi G, Mascalchi M, et al. Design, recruitment and baseline results of the ITA-LUNG trial for lung cancer screening with low dose CT. Lung Cancer 2009;64:34–40.

23. Oudkerk M, Heuvelmans MA. Screening for lung cancer by imaging: the nelson study. JBR-BTR 2013;96:163–6.

24. Midthun DE. Screening for lung cancer: the US studies. J Surg Oncol 2013;108:275–9.

Computed Tomography Screening

The International Early Lung Cancer Action Program Experience

Claudia I. Henschke, PhD, MD[a], Paolo Boffetta, MD, MPH[b],
David F. Yankelevitz, MD[a], Nasser Altorki, MD[c],*

KEYWORDS

- CT screening • Lung cancer • Assessment of benefit • Screening study design
- Diagnostic performance • Cure rate • Curability

KEY POINTS

- The Early Lung Cancer Action Project (ELCAP) was the first study of computed tomography (CT) screening for lung cancer when it started in 1992. It was designed to provide the relevant quantitative *diagnostic and prognostic* performance measures of annual CT screening using an innovative design.
- The ELCAP design recognized the profound difference between the baseline round and all subsequent rounds of annual screening and also that the annual rounds can be pooled. ELCAP also recognized that the *regimen of screening* is a critical component that determines the diagnostic and prognostic performance measures. The initial regimen was chosen to understand growth of small lung cancers, and the resulting data were used to continuously assess and update the regimen for the successor projects of the New York ELCAP and the International ELCAP (I-ELCAP).
- Key metrics of diagnostic performance are the proportion of participants diagnosed with stage I lung cancer, tumor size at diagnosis, and time from initial identification of the abnormality to treatment. The key prognostic performance measure is the *curability gain* that is achieved by early diagnosis followed by early treatment. The curability gain is defined by the proportional reduction in the case-fatality rate of lung cancer under optimal CT screening, diagnostic workup, and treatment as compared with the case-fatality rate in the absence of screening, whereby the case-fatality rate is equal to 1 minus the cure rate.

BACKGROUND

Stimulated by the technologic advances in computed tomography (CT) scanning that made it possible to image the lungs in a single breath, the Early Lung Cancer Action Project (ELCAP) was developed to assess the benefit of annual CT screening for lung cancer. The study design provided both a low-dose chest CT and a chest radiograph (CXR) to participants at high risk of lung cancer to obtain *diagnostic* information on the frequency of nodule detection and that of diagnosed lung cancers on both imaging modalities as well as prognostic information on predictors of cure and ultimately the estimated cure rate of

This report has been partially funded by a generous gift by Sonia Gardner in memory of her father Moise Lasry.
[a] Department of Radiology, Icahn School of Medicine at Mount Sinai, One Gustave L. Levy Place, New York, NY 10029, USA; [b] Department of Hematology and Oncology, Icahn School of Medicine at Mount Sinai, One Gustave L. Levy Place, New York, NY 10029, USA; [c] Department of Cardiothoracic Surgery, Weill Cornell Medical College, 525 East 68th Street, New York, NY 10065, USA
* Corresponding author.
E-mail address: nkaltork@med.cornell.edu

Thorac Surg Clin 25 (2015) 129–143
http://dx.doi.org/10.1016/j.thorsurg.2014.12.001

lung cancers diagnosed *under* screening—the screen-diagnosed cases as well as the symptom-prompted cases of lung cancer that come to attention before the next round of annual repeat screening (**Fig. 1**).[1] Critical to the diagnostic and prognostic performance is the *regimen of screening* (how to do the screening), which specified the required imaging technique, definition of a positive result, clinical workup and its timing for positive results, and the pathologic confirmation of the diagnosis.

ELCAP was started in 1992 when the initial funding was obtained. Its goal was to enroll 1000 participants, and for this it later received additional funding from a National Cancer Institute (NCI) grant.[2] The results of the baseline round of screening were reported in 1999[3] and those of annual rounds were reported in 2001.[4] ELCAP demonstrated that a high proportion of the patients with lung cancer were diagnosed in stage I with low-dose CT scans together with a shift to smaller tumor sizes, particularly on annual repeat screening. Of the participants diagnosed with stage I lung cancer in the baseline round, 83% were missed on CXRs performed at the same time[3]; thus, CXR was not provided in annual repeat screening rounds.[4]

The baseline results were widely publicized[5] and stimulated renewed public debate about the merits of screening for lung cancer. To provide further information and discuss future research projects, the ELCAP investigators organized the First International Conference on Screening for Lung Cancer in New York City in October 1999.[6] In addition to the established ELCAP investigators and others following their original paradigm,[7–11] the conference was attended by investigators from Japan who had developed their own screening programs,[12,13] representatives from the American Cancer Society, the NCI, and many other organizations, physicians, statisticians, epidemiologists, and experts in imaging and other related disciplines. The public interest in CT screening led to multiple discussions at the NCI Advisory Board meetings beginning in 1999 and led the director of the NCI to call for a Lung Cancer Progress Review Group Report[14] to establish the future research agenda. In regard to CT screening for lung cancer, the report recommended that *multiple approaches* be pursued to address all relevant questions. "Several meetings co-sponsored by NCI and the American Cancer Society have determined that several study designs in addition to a mortality endpoint-randomized trial (the gold-standard approach) are important and valid.[14]"

At the second International Conference on Screening for Lung Cancer,[6] the consensus recommendation was to pool data on CT screening from different institutions to allow for rapid assessment of its effectiveness rather than waiting for later meta-analyses of individual screening projects. To this end, a common protocol for screening was developed that was unanimously adopted at the third International Conference and that also allowed for inclusion of data from the CT screening arm of randomized controlled trials.[15,16] Subsequently a common protocol for pathology was also developed.[17]

After the initial publications[3,4] and the development of the common protocol in 2000,[16,17] ELCAP expanded to a trial of 6295 participants involving 12 institutions in the state of New York (NY-ELCAP) using the same enrollment criteria as the original ELCAP.[18] At the same time, other national and international sites expressed interest in joining ELCAP leading to the formation of the International Early Lung Cancer Action Program (I-ELCAP) collaboration in 2000, which provided further expansion to 31,567 participants who had annual CT screening and resulted in the publication of the survival benefit of CT screening.[19] According to the common I-ELCAP protocol, the research sites were permitted to set their own enrollment criteria as to age and smoking history in order to broaden the knowledge base for determining the indications for screening.[15,16] Ultimately, the goal of the ELCAP design was to provide quantitative estimates of relevant diagnostic and prognostic parameters.

DIAGNOSTIC MISSION

The ELCAP design can provide the relevant *diagnostic* information to any desired precision by

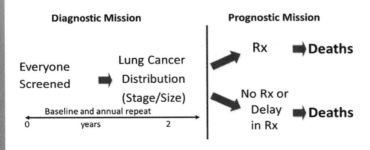

Fig. 1. In ELCAP, the diagnostic and prognostic missions are evaluated separately. The diagnostic mission is to determine the distribution of diagnosed lung cancers by relevant prognostic indicators (eg, stage and size). The prognostic mission is to determine the cure rate of the diagnosed and treated cases of lung cancer under screening. R$_x$, treatment.

providing only 2 rounds of screening: the baseline round and one single repeat round.[1] Metrics of diagnostic performance are the proportion of participants diagnosed with stage I lung cancer, tumor size at diagnosis, and time from initial identification of the abnormality to treatment. It was recognized that the *regimen of screening* is a critical component as it determines these diagnostic performance measures.

The importance of the regimen cannot be sufficiently stressed, and it was recognized that in order to remain state of the art, it must be continually updated based on advances in both knowledge and technology. The regimen defines the positive results and the workup of these positive results to limit unnecessary diagnostics while minimizing delay in diagnoses of lung cancers. The definitions may be quite different for the baseline and repeat rounds of screening. The baseline round is inherently different from all subsequent rounds of repeat screening, and it is the repeat rounds that ultimately determine the performance of any particular screening program. The ELCAP design allowed for flexibility as the recommended workup does not need to be followed but is left for shared decision making between each participant and his or her referring physician as long as the actual workup is documented.

When the original ELCAP study was developed in 1991 to 1992, the relevant clinical descriptor was the *solitary pulmonary nodule*. However, it was soon recognized that multiple nodules were being identified on CT scans; thus, this definition needed to be expanded. In the baseline round of ELCAP, a positive result was defined as identifying any noncalcified nodule regardless of size, and for annual repeat rounds it was any *new* noncalcified nodule. Using these criteria, 23% had a positive result at baseline[3] and 3% at the annual repeat round,[4] respectively. The diagnostic workup for positive results was specified, and ELCAP showed these findings could be managed with minimal use of invasive procedures. Since then, I-ELCAP has continuously updated the diagnostic regimen based on previously generated data and has incorporated the rapidly advancing technology.[16,20,21] As a result, using the I-ELCAP regimen of screening, more than 80% of the lung cancers are diagnosed while still in stage I and the tumor size is typically less than 15 mm in diameter in the baseline round.[18,19,22]

PROGNOSTIC MISSION

The *prognostic* metric used by ELCAP is the *cure rate* of cases of lung cancer diagnosed as a result of screening, which includes both screen-diagnosed cases and symptom-prompted (ie, interim) diagnosed cases. This rate is defined as the proportion of genuine cases of lung cancer curable by optimal early diagnosis followed by timely curative treatment[19] and is estimated from the Kaplan-Meier (KM) survival curve when it has reached its plateau as shown in **Fig. 2**. The benefit of screening can be measured by the *curability gain* that is achieved by the regimen, and this is defined by the proportional reduction in the fatality rate of lung cancer under optimal CT screen diagnosis and treatment as compared with the fatality rate in the absence of screening, whereby the fatality rate is equal to 1 minus the cure rate.

As it was understood that 10-year follow-up would be needed to have robust estimates of the cure rate, the ELCAP investigators sought to estimate the curability of small stage I lung cancer in the United States in comparison with larger ones. Using registry data collected by the Surveillance and End Results Registry (SEER), the estimated cure rates for stage I lung cancers that were 6 to 15 mm, 16 to 25 mm, and 26 to 30 mm in diameter that underwent resection was 75%, 69%, and 60%, respectively; for those that had no documented treatment it was 13%, 6%, and 12%, respectively.[23] Thus, the estimated curability gain for the lung cancers of 6 to 15 mm was given by [(1 − 0.13) − (1 − 0.75)]/(1 − 0.13) = 0.71 or 71%. Similarly, for tumors of 16 to 25 mm and 26 to 30 mm, it was 67% and 55%. As SEER lung cancer cases were typically diagnosed in the absence of screening at that time, the authors presumed that these estimates would provide a lower limit for those to be derived from screening studies.

After sufficient follow-up had occurred in I-ELCAP, the estimated cure rate, based on the 10-year KM lung cancer–specific survival rate, could be obtained (see **Fig. 2**).[19] It demonstrated that lung cancer survival decreased rapidly during the first 4 years after diagnosis as patients with late-stage lung cancer who were diagnosed by the screening died of their lung cancer. Others, however, whose lung cancer was diagnosed sufficiently early to undergo curative resection, did not die; thus, over time the number of deaths decrease, and as a result the survival curve begins to flatten out, eventually reaching an asymptote. The estimated cure rate in I-ELCAP was 80% (95% confidence interval [CI]: 74%–85%) for all cancers, regardless of stage, size, or treatment; it was 92% (95% CI: 88%–95%) for all patients with stage I lung cancer who underwent surgical resection within 1 month (see **Fig. 2**).[19] These cure rates translate into a 20% fatality rate for all diagnosed with lung cancer and an 8% fatality

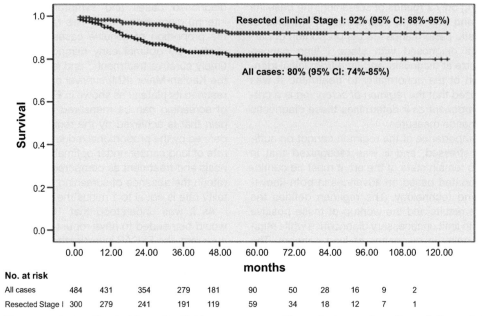

Fig. 2. The cure rate as estimated from the KM lung cancer–specific survival curve from time of diagnosis for all 484 patients who were diagnosed under the I-ELCAP regimen of screening, regardless of stage and treatment, and for those diagnosed in stage I and resected within 1 month. CI, confidence interval. (*From* The International Early Lung Cancer Action Program Investigators. Survival of patients with stage I lung cancer detected on CT screening. N Engl J Med 2006;355:1768; with permission.)

rate for those who had their stage I lung cancer resected within 1 month.

In the absence of screening, the cure rate of lung cancer, as estimated by the number of lung cancer deaths among all those diagnosed with lung cancer, has remained around 10%, essentially unchanged for decades,[24,25] so that the fatality rate in the absence of screening is 90%. Thus, the curability gain for all stages of lung cancer diagnosed under screening is $(90\% - 20\%)/90\% = 78\%$, which, as anticipated, is higher than the estimated stage I curability based on the SEER analysis of 71%.

The traditional measure of effectiveness of screening is the mortality reduction achieved under screening as compared with that in the absence of screening. This can also be determined using the I-ELCAP data if all causes of death are determined (ie, from the National Death Index [NDI]) and by comparing the deaths from lung cancer in the screening cohort with an unscreened cohort using standard statistical techniques. For this purpose, the New York State (NYS) cohort, a subcohort of I-ELCAP, was used. This cohort has documented all deaths from lung cancer and then compared them to deaths in 2 unscreened cohorts, the American Cancer Society Cancer Prevention Study II (CPS-II) cohort and the Beta-Carotene and Retinol Efficacy Trial (CARET) cohort. Using indirect standardization to

adjust for age, sex, and smoking history,[26] the comparison showed that there was a significant reduction in deaths from lung cancer in the screened NYS cohort of 36% and 64%, respectively, when compared with the unscreened CPS-II and CARET cohort. The cumulative mortality rates by year after enrollment in the NYS and CARET cohorts are shown in Fig. 3. Note that the rates remain the same over the first 4 years after enrollment. Thereafter, the cumulative mortality rate for the NYS decreases compared with CARET. As the NYS cohort provided a baseline and single annual repeat round of screening, the deaths from lung cancer then, when screening ended, started to increase 9 years after enrollment and thereafter would continue to increase, paralleling the deaths in the CARET cohort.

The lung cancer mortality in the NYS cohort was also assessed using a validated mathematical model, and it showed a mortality reduction of 46% caused by CT screening.[27] The model used the age, sex, and smoking characteristics of each NYS participant and also adjusted for the so-called healthy volunteer bias. Thus, modeling and comparison with unscreened cohorts provided a consistent estimate of mortality reduction from screening in the range of 40% to 60%.

In summary, the ELCAP design for research on the effectiveness of low-dose CT screening for lung cancer provided detailed information on the

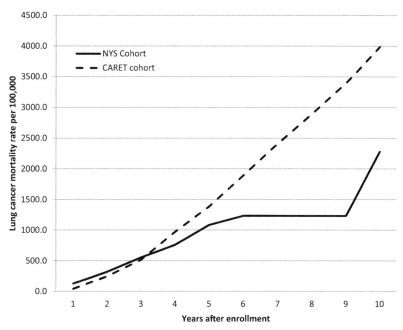

Fig. 3. Cumulative mortality rates per 100,000 person-years, separately for the CARET cohort and the NYS cohort for each year after enrollment. (*From* Henschke CI, Boffetta P, Gorlova OY, et al. Assessment of lung-cancer mortality reduction from CT screening. Lung Cancer 2011;71:330; with permission.)

diagnostic and prognostic performance of the screening process, allowed for continuous updating of the regimen of screening, and provided estimates of the cure rates of lung cancer under screening. Beyond this, an estimate of mortality reduction can also be determined.

LEAD-TIME, LENGTH, AND OVERDIAGNOSIS BIAS

Possible biases that affect the cure rate estimates obtained from the ELCAP design are *lead time, length*, and *overdiagnosis*.[28,29] *Lead time* is defined as the time by which the diagnosis under screening is advanced under screening when compared with when it is made in the absence of screening. If there is no lead time, the screening process provides no advantage. Lead-time bias exists when the cure rate is estimated using a KM survival rate before the curve reaches its asymptotic value. However, once the asymptotic value is reached, the estimates of cure rate do not have lead-time bias.[19,23]

Overdiagnosis, according to the usual definition, occurs when screening leads to diagnosis of a lung cancer and that cancer, if not diagnosed, would not have led to death. This bias can occur in 2 ways: (1) diagnosing a cancer that, even though it is a genuine life-threatening cancer, does not cause death because patients die of competing causes (eg, automobile accident, myocardial infarction),[30]

and these can be slow-growing, or (2) diagnosing a lung cancer that is genuinely indolent and does not lead to death in the absence of treatment.[31,32] Dying of competing causes of death (the first point) is partially addressed by choosing the appropriate indications for screening (eg, age, fit to undergo thoracic surgery, at least a 5- or 10-year life expectancy). The ELCAP design focuses on the second point in several ways: (1) requiring documentation of growth, at a malignant rate, for nodules less than 15 mm in size before recommendation for further invasive testing (www.IELCAP.org)[16,33]; (2) assessing the growth rates of the lung cancers diagnosed under the screening[33–35]; and (3) having an expert pathology panel review of the resected pathologic specimens[17,36–38] to confirm that the resected specimens represented genuine lung cancers. The authors also follow those participants who have documented cancer who choose not to be treated to determine their outcome with a focus on the particulars of the cancer, cell type, and CT appearance. If a certain category of diagnosed lung cancer is considered to be sufficiently slow growing based on any of the aforementioned approaches, they can be excluded from the KM survival analysis of the genuine, aggressive lung cancers. For example, typical carcinoids, as they are slow growing and not always resected, have been excluded from the published survival analysis.[19] If, however, there is still concern regarding inclusion of overdiagnosed cases, then further exclusions can be made. For example, by excluding all diagnoses of adenocarcinoma having 90% or more bronchioloalveolar features,[37] the overall cure rate in I-ELCAP was reduced from 80% to 78%.

A third bias, *length bias*, exists in the baseline round in any cancer screening program as in this round it is more likely to identify slower-growing cancers, whereas those diagnosed in repeat rounds are more typical of those diagnosed in the absence of screening. A corollary of length bias is that cancers identified in repeat rounds on average are typically smaller but also faster growing than those identified in the baseline round. Thus, length bias is addressed by analyzing the baseline and repeat rounds of screening separately.[3,4,18,19,38,39] Such an analysis will show that distribution by cancer cell types is different in the baseline round than in repeat rounds, and these differences provide valuable information as to lead time provided by the screening and also the relative aggressiveness of the different cell types. For example, small cell and squamous cell represent a much larger proportion of the cancers diagnosed in annual rounds than in the baseline round, consistent with this cell type being more aggressive than those cell types whose proportions decreased in the annual rounds.[38]

TREATMENT OF SCREEN-DIAGNOSED LUNG CANCERS

The most appropriate treatment of screen-diagnosed lung cancers that manifest as either a solid, part-solid, or nonsolid nodule is not yet fully defined. As shown in I-ELCAP, surgical intervention in the context of screening results in high cure rates and the frequency and extent of surgery for nonmalignant disease can be minimized.[40]

As CT screening typically leads to the diagnosis of small, early lung cancers, the question of limited resection in place of lobectomy is again raised, a debate that has occupied thoracic surgeons for decades. Review of the SEER database has been helpful, as it demonstrated equivalence of lobectomy and limited resection for small lung cancers less than 20 mm.[41] As the I-ELCAP data accrued, this was confirmed in the context of screening, as limited resection resulted in an equivalent survival rate as lobectomy when performed on patients with screen-detected clinical stage IA lung cancers manifesting as a solid nodule, even when controlling for potential confounders.[42] The tightly controlled prospective acquisition of data elements including comorbidities, presence of emphysema, and coronary artery calcification on the baseline CT scan and the use of the propensity scoring to create a balance of the covariates between the 2 surgical treatments supports the validity of these findings. Another important finding in both I-ELCAP surgical reports was the remarkably low surgical mortality rate of 0.9%.[40,42]

Randomized surgical trials comparing lobectomy with limited sublobar resection are ongoing in the United States and Japan; but the final results are expected in 6 to 8 years, as sufficient follow-up is needed. In the meantime, surgical techniques continue to improve.

The role of nonsurgical therapy for these lesions, such as radiation[43] or image-guided ablative therapy, is not yet well explored. Ultimately, the authors think that the course of action regarding these management decisions needs to be based on informed decision-making discussions between the patients and their physicians.

THE NATIONAL LUNG SCREENING TRIAL

Stimulated by the Lancet report in 1999[3] and the widespread interest,[5] the NCI immediately started planning the National Lung Screening Trial (NLST). The NLST used a randomized trial design that randomly assigns individuals to one of 2 study arms to test the hypothesis that CT screening would reduce lung cancer mortality over CXR screening by 20% (**Fig. 4**).[44] The NLST randomly assigned 25,000 high-risk participants to each of the 2 arms of the trial (CT vs CXR) and provided 3 rounds to each participant.[45] The NLST designers elected to use CXR screening instead of no screening in the control arm, in part, because another randomized trial, the Prostate, Lung, Colon, and Ovarian trial, which had started in 1993, was comparing CXR with no screening.[46] By 2002, in record time, the NLST was started in the United States and additional randomized trials were being started in Europe.[47,48]

Baseline screening in the NLST was completed in 2004, and 2 rounds of annual repeat screening were completed in 2004 to 2006. All participants were then followed to determine death from lung cancer, as recorded in the NDI and documented by committee review. On November 4, 2010, the NCI announced that the interim analysis of the NLST showed a statistically significant mortality lung cancer reduction of 20.3% as well as an all-cause mortality reduction that was achieved after providing 3 rounds of screening and 5 years of follow-up of the participants randomly assigned to CT or CXR.[49] As the trial had reached a statistically significant reduction in mortality with its initial goal being a 20% reduction, it was stopped and letters were sent to the participants advising them of the results and suggesting that they talk

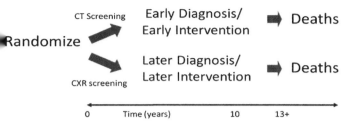

CT Screening

Early Diagnosis/
Early Intervention

➡ Deaths

CXR screening

Later Diagnosis/
Later Intervention

➡ Deaths

0   Time (years)   10   13+

Fig. 4. Design of the NLST in which participants at risk of lung cancer were randomized into 2 arms of screening for 3 rounds. As the initial diagnostic test (CXR or CT) is viewed as an intervention, all deaths from lung cancer are counted in each arm for a given period of time, regardless of the diagnostic workup and treatment, if any.

to their physician about having a CT scan. Subsequently, the final report was published in 2011, which confirmed the 20% lung cancer-specific and also an all-cause mortality reduction of 6%.[50] This study was an important confirmation of the value of CT screening for lung cancer and provided important information for a comparison of the fundamental differences in the two study designs, that of the ELCAP and the NLST.

A COMPARISON OF THE EARLY LUNG CANCER ACTION PROJECT AND NATIONAL LUNG SCREENING TRIAL STUDY DESIGNS

A fundamental difference between the ELCAP and NLST study designs is that the ELCAP design focuses on obtaining a *quantitative* estimate of the cure rate, whereas the NLST tests the *null* hypothesis that there is no difference in the cumulative mortality rates in the two arms versus the *alternative* hypothesis that there is a significant difference between the two cumulative mortality rates. It is important to understand the fundamental differences in these two approaches, and it is indeed fortunate that both studies are available, as they provide valuable information for future research efforts on assessment and implementation of screening tests and in particular blood-based, sputum, or breath tests that are being developed. Recall that as recommended by the NCI report of 2002,[14] multiple approaches should be pursued for these large public health questions.

The stark difference between providing a *quantitative estimate* and performing a test of hypothesis is often not fully appreciated. To determine a quantitative estimate, an appropriate design and strict quality-assurance measures are required at each step in the diagnostic and prognostic process, which is achieved by specifying a *regimen of screening* with all its component issues; the performance of the regimen is measured by the diagnostic distribution of the cancers and the estimated cure rate for this diagnostic distribution (see **Fig. 1**).

Hypothesis testing, on the other hand, provides a *qualitative* approach to determine whether there is or is not a *statistically significant difference*

between the *null* and the *alternative* hypothesis.[51] How is this significant difference determined? As such trials take a long time to complete, involve many participants, and are very expensive, the designers try to minimize the trial's size and duration and, thereby, the costs. They do this by choosing a cutoff for the difference in the mortality rates that is considered to be clinically important (eg, 20% in the NLST). This difference influences the study design as to the number of participants, how many rounds of screening, and length of follow-up that need to be provided.[52] All of these design parameters (significant mortality reduction, number of years of screening, and follow-up) must be determined in advance of the actual trial. But on what knowledge and data are these design parameters chosen? The mortality reduction deemed to be *significant* is set high enough to justify screening but low enough to be reliably detected using the specified study design, but it does not mean that this is the maximum reduction that can be achieved by the screening. Hypothesis testing focuses on detecting the *minimum (statistically) significant* mortality difference between the two arms so that the null hypothesis of no difference is rejected for a predetermined alpha error (the probability of rejecting the null hypothesis when it is correct) and beta error (the probability of not rejecting the null hypothesis when the alternative is correct).[51,52] If the null hypothesis is rejected, then the actual difference can be any value greater than the *minimum significant* reduction. If the hypothesis is not rejected, then the possible reasons are that minimum significant mortality difference cannot be reached by the screening; but it may also be that it could have been achieved but could not be identified because of problems in the design or implementation (eg, protocol nonadherence, that is, contamination or noncompliance, diagnostic inefficiency as reflected by a lower percentage diagnosed in stage I, larger median tumor size, and treatment inefficiencies, including delayed or suboptimal treatment or lack of any treatment).[22]

The 20% mortality reduction reported in the NLST study is almost certainly not all that could have been achieved by that design. But the fact that a significant mortality reduction was found means that factors such as protocol nonadherence and diagnostic and treatment inefficiencies did not overwhelm the benefit of the 3 rounds of CT screening. The benefit would have been larger had the trial been conducted with an alternative hypothesis requiring more than a 20% difference by using more rounds of screening, by following a strict protocol for the diagnosis workup and treatment with sufficient quality-assurance measures in place, or by using a control arm that did not also provide alternative screening. In other words, the mortality reduction demonstrated by the NLST depends on the study design and is not an inherent parameter that reflects the curability of screen-diagnosed lung cancers.

How do we reconcile the difference in the estimated cure rate of 80% or curability gain of 78% resulting from the I-ELCAP and the mortality reduction estimate of 20.3% resulting from the NLST? Clearly deaths cannot be reduced unless at least some of the participants diagnosed with lung cancer as a result of screening are cured. But why the difference in the mortality reduction reported by the NLST and the estimated cure reported by the I-ELCAP?

The outcome parameter of I-ELCAP is the cure rate achieved under screening. This quantitative rate provides a clinically relevant measure that is well understood by physicians and lay people. The rate depends on the quality of the screening regimen as measured by its diagnostic performance (eg, tumor stage and size) and the timeliness and quality of the treatment of the cancers identified by the screening as well as the frequency with which diagnoses of lung cancer are prompted by symptoms before the next annual screening.[19]

The outcome parameter of the NLST is mortality reduction, which in the clinical community seems to be less completely understood. The 20%

mortality reduction of the NLST is often misinterpreted as being the actual mortality reduction that is likely to be achieved by a CT screening program. *This interpretation is incorrect.* Specific design parameters must be reported with this result. Correctly stated, the 20.3% mortality reduction reported by the NLST resulted from a trial of 53,000+ high-risk participants who underwent CT or CXR screening for 3 years and 5 years of follow-up and had given proportions of protocol nonadherence, delay in diagnosis, and/or treatment. Thus, the mortality reduction is only meaningful in reference to that particular study's design and implementation. For example, the NLST does not provide an estimate of the mortality reduction if the regimen of screening was strictly specified and followed, if 5 or 10 rounds of screening had been provided, or when screening people of different ages and smoking histories other than those included in the study. To answer these questions, the US Preventive Services Task Force had to rely on modeling studies.[53] However, these questions can be answered by I-ELCAP–type studies, as actual data have been collected for a much wider spectrum of indications for screening.

The comparison between the mortality reduction shown by the NLST and the curability rate shown by the I-ELCAP showed that the former approach markedly underestimates the actual mortality reduction that can be provided by a program of continued CT screening. The authors proposed the ratio of the year-specific fatality rates in the two arms is a more appropriate end-point measure for randomized trials, as it provides a better estimate of the case-fatality rate (**Figs. 5** and **6**).[54–58] **Fig. 7** shows the ratio of the year-specific fatality rates in both arms of a randomized trial of screening for a cancer. Initially the rates in both arms should be essentially identical, so the ratio is close to 1. After some time, assuming screening

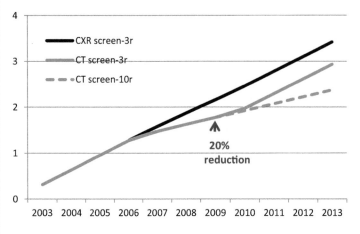

Fig. 5. Theoretic cumulative mortality rates for CT (*blue line*) and CXR (*black line*) screening for the NLST if screening is done for 3 rounds (r) or for 10 r (*dashed blue line*). As screening stopped after 3 years, the rate in the CT arm is expected to again start to increase around 2011 and parallel the rate in the CXR arm (*blue solid line*) as long as follow-up in the trial continued. However, the trial was stopped; if participants now opt for CT screening, both curves may change.

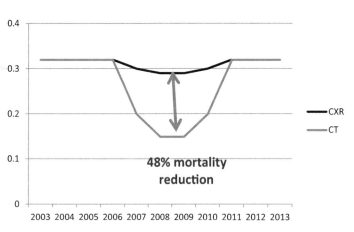

Fig. 6. The estimated year-specific fatality rate reduction for CT as compared with CXR is 48%. As there is a minimal reduction due to CXR screening, the reduction in the year-specific mortality rate per 100,000 participant-years is probably even larger if it had been compared with no screening rather than to CXR screening, as the latter has some effect.

is effective in reducing mortality, the year-specific rate in the screening arm will start to decrease, eventually reaching the lowest mortality rate provided by that screening regimen. For lung cancer, this minimum is probably reached some 7 to 10 years after the start of baseline screening as long as screening is continuous. If screening stops, the rate will again increase at the same rate it decreased until it again matches that of the control arm.

The difference between the average mortality reduction over the entire time of a randomized trial and the year-specific rate ratios has been illustrated for breast cancer screening[54] using fatality rate reduction and for prostate cancer screening using the year-specific rate reductions.[56,57] Although the overall mortality reduction was low in both of these trials, significant year-specific reductions of 55% and 67% for breast and prostate cancer, respectively, were achieved by continuous screening; but these only became evident 8 and 9 years after baseline. Both the breast and the prostate examples illustrate that cumulative mortality rates markedly underestimated the

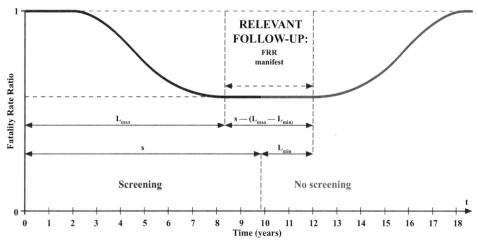

Fig. 7. Follow-up experience in a randomized controlled trial comparing screening for cancer with no screening with respect to cause-specific mortality: interrelations of parameters. At any given point in the follow-up there is a particular mortality density (MD) among the screened and the unscreened; for an interval of t to t + dt (delta t), with dC (delta C) cases expected in it, $MD_t = dC/Pdt$, where P is the size of the population. Contrasting the screened with the not screened, there is the corresponding MD ratio (MDR). This ratio is depicted as a function of time since entry into the trial. The early excess mortality among the screened is not shown, because the focus is on the intended result of reduced fatality rate (FR), quantified in terms of FR ratio (FRR). MDR coincides with FRR in a particular interval of follow-up time if the duration of screening (S) exceeds the difference between the maximum (L_{max}) and minimum (L_{min}) of the time lag from early diagnosis to the death prevented by early intervention but not by late intervention (ie, in the absence of screening). t=time in years; dt=delta t, where delta means a small increment in t; dC=delta C, where delta means a small increment in C. (*From* Henschke CI, Yankelevitz DF, Kostis WJ. CT screening for lung cancer. Semin Ultrasound CT MR 2003;24:26; with permission.)

year-specific reduction and also the reduction that would ultimately be achieved by the screening. Similarly, for lung cancer, the difference between the cumulative and annual mortality rates would only be achieved 7 years after baseline screening. Unfortunately, the drawback of using the cumulative mortality rate was not addressed in the NLST.

There are other factors that influence the results of a randomized trial so that even the year-specific rates might not provide those that could be achieved by an optimal regimen of screening. These factors include protocol nonadherence in the screening and control arms (**Fig. 8**), inaccuracies of death certificates, and diagnostic workup and/or treatment delays. These factors can obscure the true benefit, as they decrease the difference between the mortality rates in the two arms. The authors postulate that if CT screening were continued for 10 or more years using a well-defined regimen of screening with a control arm having no screening, then the maximum year-specific mortality rate in the CT arm would approach the curability as estimated by the I-ELCAP.[58]

The I-ELCAP reported a cure rate of 80%, which is equivalent to reporting a case-fatality rate of 20%. It is incorrect to equate this case-fatality rate with the mortality reduction result of the NLST. These two parameters are fundamentally different, albeit that one determinant of the reduction in that mortality rate is the reduction in the fatality rate. Once the difference between those outcome parameters is understood, it becomes clear that there is nothing inherently incompatible between the 20% reduction in mortality reported from the NLST and the curability rate of 78% reported by the I-ELCAP group. In fact, depending on the design parameters of the trial, it is possible to see differences in the mortality reduction even though the curability of the screen-detected cancers remains unchanged. For example, had the NLST been terminated 1 year earlier, as had originally been planned, it would not have shown a significant difference between the CT and CXR mortality rates. Had additional rounds of screening and a longer follow-up been performed, the mortality reduction would have been higher. The impact of the design parameters of a randomized screening trial, a stop-screening trial design, is not yet fully appreciated in the clinical domain but have been pointed out in a letter on "Understanding the Core Result of the National Lung Screening Trial" to the *New England Journal of Medicine*.[58]

This major underestimation of the reduction in fatality rate is now incorrectly being used to describe the NLST result with severe adverse consequences. Among the huge number of people at high risk for lung cancer, a large number will decide not to be screened so long as they are taught that the consequence is only a 20%

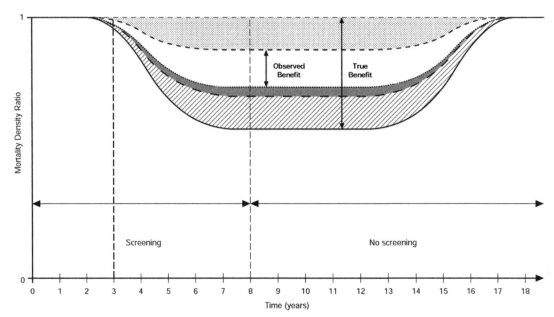

Fig. 8. Noncompliance with the screening, diagnosis, and treatment in either arm will decrease the observed benefit. When only 3 years of screening are performed, the deaths in the screening arm will again increase at the same rate they decreased so that an even smaller observed benefit may be seen. (*From* Henschke CI, Yankelevitz DF, Kostis WJ. CT screening for lung cancer. Semin Ultrasound CT MR 2003;24:27; with permission.)

reduction in death from lung cancer, as they might consider this to be too meager a benefit. If those people knew that perhaps 3 of 4 otherwise incurable lung cancers could be cured when diagnosed under the screening, surely the conversation about risks and benefits would be dramatically different; the number of people choosing to be screened, leading to lives that would be saved, would be enormous.

Guideline organizations relied on that relative mortality reduction found in NLST to define the benefit associated with screening and ultimately endorsed screening.[59] However, when it came to explaining that result to people interested in screening, they thought it necessary to move the discussion away from the population measure of mortality and instead to discuss the clinical concept of reduction provided by case-fatality. So although no attempt was made to measure case-fatality reduction as an end point in the NLST, it was recognized by the guideline organizations that when talking to potential participants to be screened, they needed to use statements about case-fatality.[59]

Cost-effectiveness of screening has been studied both in the context of the I-ELCAP[60] and for participants aged 65 years and older who are covered by the Centers for Medicare and Medicaid Services.[61]

INTERNATIONAL EARLY LUNG CANCER ACTION PROJECT IN THE FUTURE

The I-ELCAP presents a new paradigm that addresses the NCI's 2002 recommendations for pursuit of multiple approaches to address all relevant questions[14] and the recommendations by the Institute of Medicine (IOM) Roundtable on Evidence-Based Medicine[62] from the National Academy of Sciences that a "new clinical paradigm be developed that takes better advantage of data generated in the course of healthcare delivery which would speed and improve the development of evidence for real-world decision making."

The I-ELCAP is a cohort study for the assessment of CT screening for lung cancer, but it can also be used for other purposes. To date, the I-ELCAP investigators have recruited more than 66,000 participants worldwide who are 40 years of age or older and are either current smokers, former smokers, never smokers, or have occupational exposure to known carcinogens. In this context, the I-ELCAP investigators have provided the initial evidence for moving forward with further screening studies and also stimulated development of entirely new research domains, including computer-assisted 3-dimensional nodule growth

analysis,[31,63–66] smoking cessation in the context of screening[67–69] measuring extent of emphysema,[70] quantifying coronary calcium on low-dose scans as a measure of cardiac disease,[71–74] quantifying breast density on low-dose CT,[75] and evaluating early interstitial lung disease.[16]

The approach to treatment of small, early lung cancers is now being critically assessed as lung-tissue sparing becomes more important because patients are cured of their first lung cancer with increased frequency but are at high risk of developing additional primaries requiring further resection. Innovative approaches to more rapid assessment of alternative treatments are needed. The ELCAP Web-based management system[76] provides the necessary infrastructure for performing such trials and has the advantage of having been well tested by the collaborative team and can easily add additional users.

SUMMARY

The authors have suggested that cancer screening programs can be evaluated based on studies measuring relevant diagnostic parameters of the disease, such as size and stage in lung cancer, and relevant prognostic parameters, such as the cure rate or its complement, case-fatality rate. The ELCAP study design has, thus, presented a challenge to the traditional view of the supremacy of the randomized trial in the evaluation of the effectiveness of screening. But even in 2002,[12] the NCI report recommended that multiple approaches be pursued to address all relevant questions; the IOM Roundtable on Evidence-Based Medicine[62] from the National Academy of Sciences suggested that a "new clinical paradigm be developed that takes better advantage of data generated in the course of healthcare delivery which would speed and improve the development of evidence for real-world decision making."

The ELCAP approach was designed to provide data in screening for a cancer in a clinical setting that can be readily translated into a widespread screening program. It provided a protocol that allowed data generated in the course of health care delivery to be collected, pooled, and analyzed so that the regimen of screening could be continually updated. The IOM report[62] also recognized the limitations of the randomized trial, stating that "as useful as it is under the right circumstances, [it] takes too much time, is too expensive, and is fraught with questions of generalizability." The IOM report also addressed the need to better characterize the range of alternatives to the randomized trial (eg, quasi-experimental trials) and their applications and implications. The authors would suggest that the ELCAP design and its protocol, which provides for pooling of data on a global basis, provides for such a new paradigm.

Randomized trials, when properly designed and implemented, provide important evidence for testing the hypothesis of a mortality reduction from preventive and screening efforts. But problems encountered by the use of cumulative mortality reduction as a measure of effectiveness in randomized trials have highlighted the problems resulting from the dependence of the outcome measure of such a trial on the number of rounds of screening that are provided and on the lack of focus on the time when the mortality reduction is expected to become evident. Thus, randomized trials have a propensity to lead to incorrect negative trial results when not properly designed and, when positive (ie, the null hypothesis is rejected), to lead to an underestimate of the mortality reduction from screening.[53–58] In addition, the factors affecting the estimates, such as protocol nonadherence, must also be addressed. Because of their experimental design, randomized trials cannot address the full spectrum of effects of a complex diagnostic process followed by treatment that aims to modify the natural history of a disease. Even in the best-designed randomized trial, ethical considerations require the investigators to modify the control arm. For example, instead of the control arm of the NLST being no screening, CXR screening was used, but it probably does have some benefit, thus, decreasing the difference between the mortality rates of the two arms (see **Fig. 8**). The impact of these design factors needs to be clearly stated, and estimates of their influence should be provided when presenting results of these trials.

The NLST was initiated after the ELCAP report in 1999, which was sufficiently compelling to awaken interest in screening for lung cancer. During the 8 years of conducting the trial, the NLST has cost more than $300 million to provide a qualitatively correct answer but this has unfortunately been misinterpreted as to its meaning. Throughout the past decade, the 90% death rate from lung cancer in the unscreened population has continued. Public funds for nonrandomized screening studies were nearly impossible to obtain because of the commitment to the dominant paradigm of the randomized trial. The authors think that the I-ELCAP and NLST story provides a strong argument for relevant agencies to reconsider the priorities for the public funding of studies aimed at evaluating the effectiveness of screening and other medical trials. To achieve this end, a dialogue should be encouraged between the investigators involved in the different types of studies in order to secure the maximum benefit from all approaches and, thereby, create a balanced funding portfolio for different designs in support of research on cancer screening.

REFERENCES

1. Henschke CI, Miettinen OS, Yankelevitz DF, et al. Radiographic screening for cancer: proposed paradigm for requisite research. Clin Imaging 1994;18: 16–20.
2. Henschke CI. Early detection and diagnosis of lung cancer using CT. National Cancer Institute Investigator initiated grant (R01-CA-63393).
3. Henschke CI, McCauley DI, Yankelevitz DF, et al. Early Lung Cancer Action Project: overall design and findings from baseline screening. Lancet 1999;354:99–105.
4. Henschke CI, Naidich DP, Yankelevitz DF, et al. Early Lung Cancer Action Project: preliminary findings on annual repeat screening. Cancer 2001;92:153–9.
5. Grady D. CAT scan process could cut deaths from lung cancer. Small tumors detected. New York Times 1999;1.
6. International Early Lung Cancer Action Program Conferences and Consensus Statements. Available at: http://events.ielcap.org/conferences/past. Accessed February 13, 2015.
7. Diederich S, Wormanns D, Semik M, et al. Screening for early lung cancer with low-dose spiral CT: prevalence in 817 asymptomatic smokers. Radiology 2002;222:773–81.
8. Shaham D, Breuer R, Copel L, et al. Computed tomography screening for lung cancer: applicability of an international protocol in a single-institution environment. Clin Lung Cancer 2006;7:262–7.
9. Bastarrika G, Garcia-Velloso MJ, Lozano MD, et al. Early lung cancer detection with spiral computed tomography and positron emission tomography. Am J Respir Crit Care Med 2005;171:1378–83.
10. Chirikos TN, Hazelton T, Tockman M, et al. Screening for lung cancer with CT: a preliminary cost-effectiveness analysis. Chest 2002;121:1507–14.
11. Swensen SJ, Jett JR, Sloan JA, et al. Screening for lung cancer with low-dose spiral computed tomography. Am J Respir Crit Care Med 2002;165:508–13.
12. Sone S, Li F, Yang ZG, et al. Results of three-year mass screening programme for lung cancer using mobile low-dose spiral computed tomography scanner. Br J Cancer 2001;84:25–32.
13. Sobue T, Moriyama N, Kaneko M, et al. Screening for lung cancer with low-dose helical computed tomography: anti-lung cancer association project. J Clin Oncol 2002;20:911–20.
14. Lung Cancer Progress Review Group Report 2001. Chantilly (VA): National Cancer Institute; 2001. Available at: http://planning.cancer.gov/library/2001lung.pdf. Accessed February 13, 2015.

15. Henschke CI, Yankelevitz DF, Smith JP, et al. Screening for lung cancer: the Early Lung Cancer Action approach. Lung Cancer 2002;35:143–8.

16. International Early Lung Cancer Action Program protocol. Available at: http://www.ielcap.org/sites/default/files/I-ELCAP%20protocol-v21-3-1-14.pdf. Accessed February 13, 2015.

17. Vazquez M, Flieder D, Travis W, et al. Early Lung Cancer Action Project pathology protocol. Lung Cancer 2003;39:231–2. Available at: http://www.ielcap.org/sites/default/files/pathology_protocol.pdf. Accessed February 13, 2015.

18. New York Early Lung Cancer Action Project Investigators. CT Screening for lung cancer: diagnoses resulting from the New York Early Lung Cancer Action Project. Radiology 2007;243:239–49.

19. International Early Lung Cancer Investigators. Survival of patients with stage I lung cancer detected on CT screening. N Engl J Med 2006;355:1763–71.

20. Henschke CI, Yankelevitz DF, Naidich DP, et al. CT screening for lung cancer: suspiciousness of nodules according to size on baseline scans. Radiology 2004;231:164–8.

21. Henschke CI, Yip R, Yankelevitz DF, et al, for the I-ELCAP Investigators. Definition of a positive test result in computed tomography screening for lung cancer: a cohort study. Ann Intern Med 2013;158: 246–52.

22. International Early Lung Cancer Action Program Investigators, Yip R, Henschke CI, et al. The impact of the regimen of screening on lung cancer cure: a comparison of I-ELCAP and NLST. Eur J Cancer Prev 2014. [Epub ahead of print].

23. Henschke CI, Wisnivesky JP, Yankelevitz DF, et al. Screen-diagnosed small stage I cancers of the lung: genuineness and curability. Lung Cancer 2003;39:327–30.

24. American Cancer Society. Statistics 2006; cancer facts and figures. Available at: http://www.cancer.org/acs/groups/content/@nho/documents/document/caff2006pwsecuredpdf.pdf. Accessed February 13, 2015.

25. Raz DJ, Zell JA, Ou SH, et al. Natural history of stage I non-small cell lung cancer. Chest 2007;132:193–8.

26. Henschke CI, Boffetta P, Gorlova OY, et al. Assessment of lung-cancer mortality reduction from CT screening. Lung Cancer 2011;71:328–32.

27. Foy M, Yip R, Chen X, et al. Modeling the mortality reduction due to CT screening for lung cancer. Cancer 2011;117:2703–8.

28. Hutchinson GB, Shapiro S. Lead time gained by diagnostic screening for breast cancer. J Natl Cancer Inst 1968;41:665–81.

29. Morrison AS. The effects of early treatment, lead time and length bias on the mortality experienced by cases detected by screening. Int J Epidemiol 1982;11:261–7.

30. Henschke CI, Yip R, Yankelevitz DF, et al. CT screening for lung cancer: competing causes of death. Clin Lung Cancer 2006;7:323–5.

31. Kostis WJ, Yankelevitz DF, Reeves AP, et al. Small pulmonary nodules: reproducibility of three-dimensional volumetric measurement and estimation of time to follow-up CT. Radiology 2004;231: 446–52.

32. Yankelevitz DF, Kostis WF, Henschke CI, et al. Overdiagnosis in chest radiographic screening for lung carcinoma: frequency. Cancer 2003;97:1271–5.

33. Henschke CI, Shaham D, Yankelevitz DF, et al. CT Screening for lung cancer: significance of diagnoses in the baseline cycle of screening. Clin Imaging 2006;30:11–5.

34. Henschke CI, Yankelevitz DF, Yip R, et al, Writing Committee for the I-ELCAP Investigators. Lung cancers diagnosed by annual CT screening: volume doubling times. Radiology 2012;263:578–83.

35. Xu DM, Yip R, Smith JP, et al, Writing Committee for the I-ELCAP Investigators. Retrospective review of lung cancers diagnosed in annual rounds of CT screening. AJR Am J Roentgenol 2014;203(5):965–72.

36. Flieder DB, Vazquez M, Carter D, et al. Pathologic findings of lung tumors diagnosed on baseline CT screening. Am J Surg Pathol 2006;30:606–13.

37. Vazquez M, Carter D, Brambilla E, et al. Solitary and multiple resected adenocarcinomas after CT screening for lung cancer: histopathologic features and their prognostic implications. Lung Cancer 2009;64:148–54.

38. Carter D, Vazquez M, Flieder DB, et al, ELCAP and NY-ELCAP Investigators. Comparison of pathologic findings of baseline and annual repeat cancers diagnosed on CT screening. Lung Cancer 2007;56:193–9.

39. Austin JJ, Yip R, D-Souza BM, et al, for the I-ELCAP Investigators. Small-cell carcinoma of the lung detected by CT screening: stage distribution and curability. Lung Cancer 2012;76:339–43.

40. Flores R, Bauer T, Aye R, et al, for the I-ELCAP Investigators. Balancing curability and unnecessary surgery in the context of CT screening for lung cancer. J Thorac Cardiovasc Surg 2014;147: 1619–26.

41. Wisnivesky JP, Henschke CI, Swanson S, et al. Limited resection for the treatment of patients with stage IA lung cancer. Ann Surg 2010;251:550–4.

42. Altorki N, Yip R, Hanaoka T, et al, for the I-ELCAP Investigators. Sub-lobar resection is equivalent to lobectomy for clinical stage IA lung cancer in solid nodules. J Thorac Cardiovasc Surg 2014;147:754–62 [discussion: 762–4].

43. Buckstein M, Yip R, Yankelevitz D, et al. Radiation therapy for stage I lung cancer detected on computed tomography screening: results from the International Lung Cancer Action Program. J Radiat Oncol 2014;251:1–5.

44. Aberle DR, Black WC, Goldin JG, et al. Contemporary screening for the detection of lung cancer protocol [NLST], 10 May 2002. American College of Radiology Imaging Network; 2003 (ACRIN sharp6654). Available at: http://www.acrin.org/6654_protocol.aspx. Accessed February 13, 2015.

45. National Lung Screening Trial Research Team. The National Lung Screening Trial: overview and study design. Radiology 2011;258:243–53.

46. Prorok PC, Andriole GL, Bresalier RS, et al. Design of the Prostate, Lung, Colorectal and Ovarian (PLCO) cancer screening trial. Control Clin Trials 2000;21:2735–3098.

47. Van Iersel CA, de Koning JH, Draisma G, et al. Risk-based selection from the general population in a screening trial (NELSON). Int J Cancer 2007;12:868–74.

48. Pastorino U, Bellomi M, Landoni E, et al. Early lung-cancer detection with spiral CT and positron emission tomography in heavy smokers. Lancet 2003;362:593–7.

49. Lung cancer screening trial results show mortality benefit with low-dose CT. 2010. Available at: http://www.cancer.gov/newscenter/newsfromnci/2010/NLSTresultsRelease. Accessed February 13, 2015.

50. National Lung Screening Trial Research Team. Reduced lung-cancer mortality with low-dose computed tomographic screening. N Engl J Med 2011;365:395–409.

51. Prorok PC, Marcus PM. Cancer screening trials: nuts and bolts. Semin Oncol 2010;37:216–23.

52. Connor RJ, Eng D, Prorok PC. Issues in the mortality analysis of randomized controlled trials for cancer screening. Control Clin Trials 1994;15:81–99.

53. Screening for lung cancer. United States Preventive Services Task Force. Available at: http://www.uspreventiveservicestaskforce.org/uspstf/uspslung.htm. Accessed February 13, 2015.

54. Miettinen OS, Henschke CI, Pasmantier MW, et al. Mammographic screening: no reliable supporting evidence? Lancet 2002;359:404–5.

55. I-ELCAP Investigators. An update of CT screening for lung cancer. Semin Ultrasound CT MR 2005;26:348–56.

56. Hanley JA. Analysis of mortality data from cancer screening studies: looking in the right window. Epidemiology 2005;16:786–90.

57. Hanley JA. Mortality reductions produced by sustained prostate cancer screening have been underestimated. J Med Screen 2010;17:147–51.

58. Yankelevitz DF, Smith JP. Understanding the core result of the National Lung Screening Trial. N Engl J Med 2013;368:1460–1 [Erratum appears in N Engl J Med 2013;368:1757].

59. Bach PB, Mirkin JN, Oliver TK, et al. Benefits and harms of CT screening for lung cancer: a systematic review. JAMA 2012;307:2418–29.

60. Wisnivesky JP, Mushlin A, Sicherman N, et al. Cost-effectiveness of baseline low-dose CT screening for lung cancer: preliminary results. Chest 2003;124:614–21.

61. Pyenson B, Henschke CI, Yankelevitz DF, et al. Offering lung cancer screening to high-risk Medicare beneficiaries saves lives and is cost effective: an actuarial analysis. Am Health Drug Benefits 2014;7:272–82.

62. Olsen LA, Aisner D, McGinnis JM, editors. The Learning Healthcare System: workshop summary of the Institute of Medicine Roundtable on Evidence-Based Medicine. Washington, DC: National Academy Press(US); 2007. p. 4–10. ISBN: 978-0-309-103-00. [report].

63. Yankelevitz DF, Gupta R, Zhao B, et al. Repeat CT scanning for evaluation of small pulmonary nodules: preliminary results. Radiology 1999;212:561–6.

64. Yankelevitz DF, Reeves A, Kostis W, et al. Determination of malignancy in small pulmonary nodules based on volumetrically determined growth rates: preliminary results. Radiology 2000;217:251–6.

65. Reeves A, Chan A, Yankelevitz D, et al. On measuring the change in size of pulmonary nodules. IEEE Trans Med Imaging 2006;25:433–50.

66. Henschke CI, Yankelevitz DF, Yip R, et al, As the Writing Committee for the I-ELCAP Investigators. Lung cancers diagnosed by annual CT screening: volume doubling times. Radiology 2012;76:339–43.

67. Ostroff J, Buckshee N, Mancuso CA, et al. Smoking cessation: an unexpected benefit of screening CT for detection of early lung cancer. Prev Med 2001;33:613–21.

68. Anderson CM, Yip R, Henschke CI, et al. Smoking cessation and relapse during a lung cancer screening program. Cancer Epidemiol Biomarkers Prev 2009;18:3476–83.

69. Ostroff JS, Henschke CI, Yip R, et al. Smoking cessation among current smokers following enrollment in a lung cancer screening program. Cancer Epidemiology, Biomarkers and Prevention 2015, in press.

70. Zulueta J, Wisnivesky JP, Henschke CI, et al. Scoring of emphysema detected on low-dose CT predicts death from chronic obstructive pulmonary disease and lung cancer. Chest 2012;141:1216–23.

71. Shemesh J, Henschke CI, Yip R, et al. Detection of coronary artery calcification by age and gender on low-dose CT screening for lung cancer. Clin Imaging 2006;30:181–5.

72. Shemesh J, Henschke CI, Shaham D, et al. Ordinal scoring of coronary artery calcifications on low-dose CT scans of the chest predicts deaths from cardiovascular disease. Radiology 2010;257:541–8.

73. Yankelevitz DF, Henschke CI, Yip R, et al, FAMRI-IELCAP Investigators. Secondhand tobacco smoke

in never smokers is a significant risk factor for coronary artery calcification. JACC Cardiovasc Imaging 2013;6:651–7.

74. Hecht HS, de Siqueira ME, Cham M, et al. Low versus standard dose coronary artery calcium scanning. Eur Heart J Cardiovasc Imaging 2014. [Epub ahead of print].

75. Salvatore M, Margolies L, Kale M, et al. Breast density: comparison of chest CT with mammography. Radiology 2014;270(1):67–73.

76. Reeves AP, Kostis WJ, Yankelevitz DF, et al. A web-based data system for multi-institutional research studies on lung cancer. Radiologic Society of North America Scientific Session. Chicago, November 27, 2001.

Results of the National Lung Cancer Screening Trial: Where Are We Now?

Neel P. Chudgar, MD, Peter R. Bucciarelli, MD,
Elizabeth M. Jeffries, Nabil P. Rizk, MD, Bernard J. Park, MD,
Prasad S. Adusumilli, MD, David R. Jones, MD*

KEYWORDS

- Lung cancer • Screening • Low-dose CT • NLST

KEY POINTS

- In 2011, the National Lung Screening Trial (NLST) demonstrated a 20% reduction in disease-specific mortality using low-dose CT (LDCT) screening of a high-risk population compared with chest radiography (CXR).
- The United States Preventive Services Task Force (USPSTF) recommends screening high-risk individuals aged 55 to 80 years with annual LDCT.
- In November 2014, the Centers for Medicare & Medicaid Services (CMS) proposed to allow once-yearly screening for lung cancer with low dose computed tomography (LDCT) in appropriately selected patients.

INTRODUCTION

Screening for cancers in selected patient populations has become a well-established element of health care in the United States.[1] The most common cancers, in order of decreasing incidence, are prostate, breast, lung, and colorectal.[2] The treatment of breast and colorectal cancer has benefited from the widespread adoption of screening recommendations, whereas the treatment of prostate cancer, for which the USPSTF does not have screening recommendations (Table 1), has used the prostate-specific antigen test and digital rectal examination for screening for many years.[3] As a result, 93% of prostate cancers are diagnosed at a local or regional stage, and 61% of breast cancers are diagnosed at a local stage. These screening practices contribute to the high overall 5-year survival rates for prostate and breast cancer: 99.7% and 90.3%, respectively.[4] The incidence of colorectal cancer has been decreasing by 2% to 3% per year during the past 15 years, whereas the rate of screening for colorectal cancer among average-risk patients has simultaneously grown to more than 60%.[5]

Lung cancer remains the leading cause of cancer death for both men and women in the United States, and it is expected to kill approximately 86,930 men and 72,330 women in 2014 in the United States alone.[2] Yet, there is no broadly adopted screening protocol for patients at high risk of developing lung cancer. More than 400,000 people in the United States have a history of lung cancer, and an estimated 224,210 new cases will be diagnosed in 2014.[4] Early-stage lung cancers often develop asymptomatically or

Conflicts of Interest/Disclosure Statement: All authors declare no conflicts of interest and have no disclosures to make.
Thoracic Service, Department of Surgery, Memorial Sloan Kettering Cancer Center, 1275 York Avenue, New York, NY 10065, USA
* Corresponding author. Thoracic Service, Department of Surgery, Memorial Sloan Kettering Cancer Center, 1275 York Avenue, Box 7, New York, NY 10065.
E-mail address: jonesd2@mskcc.org

Thorac Surg Clin 25 (2015) 145–153
http://dx.doi.org/10.1016/j.thorsurg.2014.11.002
1547-4127/15/$ – see front matter © 2015 Elsevier Inc. All rights reserved.

Table 1
US Preventive Service Task Force screening recommendations

Cancer	Specified Population	Screening Recommendation	Grade
Prostate	NA	No screening recommended	D
Breast	Women aged ≥40 y	Mammography every 1–2 y, with or without BSE	B
Colon	Adults aged 50–75 y	FOBT annually OR flexible sigmoidoscopy with FOBT every 3 y OR colonoscopy every 10 y	A
Cervical	Women aged 21–65 y	Papanicolaou smear every 3 y	A
	Women aged 30–65 y wanting to lengthen screening interval	Papanicolaou smear and HPV testing every 5 y	

Grade A: the USPSTF recommends the service. There is high certainty that the net benefit is substantial.
   Grade B: the USPSTF recommends the service. There is high certainty that the net benefit is moderate or there is moderate certainty that the net benefit is moderate to substantial.
   Grade D: the USPSTF recommends against the service. There is moderate or high certainty that the service has no net benefit or that the harms outweigh the benefits.
   Abbreviations: BSE, breast self-examination; FOBT, fecal occult blood testing; HPV, human papilloma virus; NA, not applicable.
   Data from Recommendations. U.S. Preventive Services Task Force. 2014. Available at: http://www.uspreventiveservices taskforce.org/Page/Name/recommendations. Accessed November 19, 2014.

with nonspecific symptoms. This feature, combined with the lack of an established screening protocol, plays a role in 57% of non–small cell lung cancers diagnosed at an advanced stage,[4] which carry a dismal 5-year survival rate of only 4%.[2] Alternatively, lung cancers diagnosed at an early stage have a much better 5-year survival rate, of 53.5%, with 68% of early-stage lung cancers amenable to surgical resection.[4] Comparatively, only 8% of stage III and IV tumors were operatively managed in 2011.[4] Thus, there is great potential to reduce mortality by establishing an early detection program for lung cancer.

Several previous initiatives to assess the feasibility of early detection in individuals with the highest risk of developing lung cancer have been completed. Early trials investigating the utility of CXR and sputum cytology as screening modalities were unable to demonstrate a mortality benefit.[6–9]

As imaging technologies have advanced, attention has turned to CT as a modality for lung cancer screening.[10–13] The Early Lung Cancer Action Project, for instance, published a series of 1000 patients who underwent LDCT screening and suggested that this modality was superior to CXR for detecting malignant nodules at early stages (**Fig. 1**). Although these initial findings were promising, this study was not designed to include a control arm for comparison, necessitating further research.[10] In 2011, a NLST research group published results from the largest-to-date, randomized, multicenter study, which included more than 50,000 patients and tested the utility of LDCT versus conventional CXR for lung cancer screening In high-risk patients. This well-developed and rigorous study observed a 20% decrease in disease-specific mortality in the LDCT group.[14,15] Stated differently, 3 deaths were averted for every

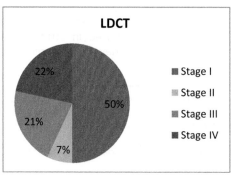
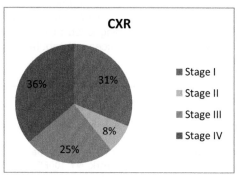

Fig. 1. Diagnoses, by stage, for LDCT and CXR. (*Data from* Aberle DR, Adams AM, Berg CD, et al. Reduced lung-cancer mortality with low-dose computed tomographic screening. N Engl J Med 2011;365(5):395–409.)

1000 study participants screened annually during a 3-year period.[16] The NLST was a landmark step forward toward the goal of early detection of lung cancer in high-risk patients.

NATIONAL LUNG SCREENING TRIAL
Trial Design and Methods

The NLST was a multicenter, randomized controlled trial funded by the National Cancer Institute that compared LDCT and CXR as screening modalities in patients considered at high risk of developing lung cancer. The study enrolled 53,454 participants. The primary outcome was lung cancer mortality, which was compared between the 2 arms of the trial. Secondary outcomes included incidence of lung cancer and causes of death other than lung cancer. Participants were enrolled between August 2002 and April 2004 at 33 centers across the Unites States, and data were captured through December 31, 2009. Inclusion criteria were age between 55 and 74 years and a minimum smoking history of 30 pack-years (former smokers who quit smoking within 15 years of study enrollment were also included). Patients who reported a previous diagnosis of lung cancer, weight loss, or hemoptysis or who had undergone chest CT during the 18 months before enrollment were excluded. A total of 26,722 individuals were randomized to receive LDCT, and 26,732 were randomized to receive CXR. Participants in the LDCT group received a baseline CT scan, denoted as T0, and 2 subsequent annual LDCT scans, denoted as T1 and T2. The average effective dose of each LDCT scan was 1.5 mSv, which is less than 25% of the average effective radiation dose of a diagnostic chest CT scan.[17] Subjects in the CXR group received a single-view posteroanterior CXR at baseline, followed by 2 annual screening CXRs.[15] To ensure standardization of imaging and interpretation, radiologists and technologists who participated in the study were trained in accordance with NLST protocols. Positive CT findings included noncalcified nodules at least 4 mm in size, pleural effusions, and lymphadenopathy. Similarly, any noncalcified nodule or mass on CXR was considered a positive finding. Follow-up of positive findings was left to the discretion of the interpreting team, although guidelines were developed and made available. Stable nodules were defined as nodules that remained unchanged through all 3 rounds of LDCT screening.[14]

Results

Compliance remained high throughout the trial, with more than 90% of patients in each group completing the screening protocol. In total, 24% of patients in the LDCT group had positive screening results compared with 7% in the CXR group. Positive scans, by screening interval, are shown in **Table 2**.[14] As expected, there were fewer positive scans at the T2 interval, because some nodules followed through the course of the study were deemed stable. Overall, 39.1% of patients in the LDCT group and 16.0% of patients in the CXR group had at least 1 positive screen during the trial. Abnormalities that were not suspicious for lung cancer were found in 7.5% of subjects in the LDCT group and 2% of subjects in the CXR group.[14]

Among the patients with a positive screening result, 1060 lung cancers were diagnosed in the LDCT group compared with 941 in the CXR group. There were 356 deaths in the LDCT group and 443 in the CXR group. These findings represent a 20% decrease in disease-specific mortality in the LDCT group. All-cause mortality was 6.7% lower in the LDCT group than in the CXR group. False-positive rates were 96.4% in the LDCT group and 95.4% in the CXR group.[14] The sensitivity and specificity of each intervention, by screening interval, are shown in **Table 3**. LDCT had a higher sensitivity for identifying lesions compared with CXR, but LDCT had a lower specificity.[18,19]

Table 2
Positive screens per screening interval

| Interval | LDCT | | CXR | |
	Positive (%)	Negative[a]	Positive (%)	Negative
T0	7191 (27.3)	19,118	2387 (9.2)	23,648
T1	6901 (27.9)	17,814	1482 (6.2)	22,607
T2	4054 (16.8)	20,048	1174 (5.0)	22,172

[a] Negative, clinically significant abnormality not suspicious for lung cancer, minor abnormality, normal.
   Data from Aberle DR, Adams AM, Berg CD, et al. Reduced lung-cancer mortality with low-dose computed tomographic screening. N Engl J Med 2011;365(5):395–409.

Table 3
Sensitivity and specificity per screening interval

Interval	Low-dose CT		Chest Radiography	
	Sensitivity	Specificity	Sensitivity	Specificity
T0	93.8	73.4	73.5	91.3
T1	94.4	72.6	59.6	94.1
T2	93.0	83.9	63.9	95.3

Data are percentages.
Data from Aberle DR, DeMello S, Berg CD, et al. Results of the two incidence screenings in the national lung screening trial. N Engl J Med 2013;369(10):920–31; and Church TR, Black WC, Aberle DR, et al. Results of initial low-dose computed tomographic screening for lung cancer. N Engl J Med 2013;368(21):1980–91.

The study found that approximately 90% of patients with a positive finding at the T0 interval underwent additional work-up, which typically involved further imaging and less frequently involved invasive procedures, including percutaneous biopsy, bronchoscopy, or a surgical procedure. Complications occurred in 1.4% of patients in the LDCT group and 1.6% of patients in the CXR group. Most of the complications were in patients with a confirmed diagnosis of lung cancer.[14] The reduction in lung cancer mortality observed in the LDCT group likely resulted from the increased diagnosis of early-stage lung cancers—57% of cancers diagnosed in the LDCT group were stage I or II tumors; in the CXR group, only 39% of cancers were diagnosed at similarly early stages. At the T1 screening interval, the CXR group had a higher percentage (59.1%) of disseminated cancers at diagnosis compared with the LDCT group (31.1%).[18] Overall, in the NLST study, there was a 2.7-fold increase in the diagnosis of lung cancer with LDCT screening compared with CXR screening.[18]

COMPLICATIONS AND CONCERNS
Potential Harms of Low-Dose CT Screening

As listed in **Box 1**, there are several concerns associated with the broad implementation of LDCT for lung cancer screening. One of the most apparent potential harms is false-positive results, which occur with a high incidence. False-positive results can increase anxiety in patients, prompting further diagnostic testing and carrying additional risks.[17] Of the 17,053 patients in the NLST who received a positive screening result without subsequent confirmation of lung cancer, 457 (2.7%) underwent 1 or more invasive procedures (mediastinoscopy, thoracoscopy, thoracotomy, bronchoscopy, or needle biopsy), with 9.6% of these patients experiencing at least 1 complication.[14] The incidence of invasive procedures among these patients can be contrasted with that among patients undergoing screening for breast cancer: 7% to 10% of biopsies among patients screened for breast cancer yielded nonmalignant diagnoses through 10 years of annual screening.[20]

Overdiagnosis occurs when a cancer is diagnosed that would otherwise remain clinically insignificant.[14] Such patients are then subjected to further diagnostic and therapeutic interventions, which carry risk. The extent of overdiagnosis in the NLST cannot be determined yet, because further follow-up is required.[17] Screening guidelines for other tumors play a similar role in their overdiagnosis. An analysis of Surveillance, Epidemiology, and End Results Program data found that, in 2008, 31% of breast cancers were overdiagnosed after screening mammography.[21]

With increasing exposure to ionizing radiation from screening or diagnostic CT scans, the risk of radiation-induced cancers also must be weighed.[18] A diagnostic chest CT provides approximately 8 mSv of radiation, and a positron emission tomography/CT delivers approximately 14 mSv.[17] Although the level of radiation of a screening CT is much lower, at 1.5 mSv, this dose cannot be considered negligible in the context of repeated examinations. Annual screening for lung cancer by LDCT could result in a 0.2% to 0.85% increased lifetime risk of developing cancer, depending on

Box 1
Concerns associated with low-dose CT screening for lung cancer

False-positive results

Nonstandardized follow-up

Overdiagnosis

Radiation exposure

Cost

Nonadherence

age, gender, and smoking status.[22] Overall, as many as 1.5% to 2% of cancers in the United States are estimated the result of radiation from current imaging use.[23]

Limitations of the National Lung Screening Trial

Although the NLST was able to establish a significant associated decrease in lung cancer–specific mortality, the investigators note several caveats to the global application of their findings. First, the study was performed at 33 medical centers with highly trained personnel and specialized physicians. Applicability at the community level is thus a concern, because image interpretation, follow-up, and management can vary. Second, patients subjected to screening within the community likewise may not reflect those recruited for the NLST. In what is recognized as the *healthy volunteer effect*, a bias toward findings with better outcomes may result from study participants. Because the screenings for this study took place between 2002 and 2007, the investigators note that newer-generation CT scanners in use now may lead to more positive scans. Last, the study showed a higher positive predictive value for lesions diagnosed at the T2 interval. Thus, continuing past 3 annual screenings may result in a greater reduction in mortality than the results of this study have demonstrated.[14,18,19]

In response to the large number of false-positive results and the low positive predictive value observed, the study investigators also discuss refining the screening protocols. They note a low incidence of lung cancer in subjects between 55 and 59 years of age and suggest increasing the minimum age requirement for screening. Because nodule size also correlated with likelihood of cancer, they suggest establishing predictive algorithms to better direct the follow-up for lesions found.[18] The CT appearance of nodules in terms of percentage of solid component and histologic appearance can also be included in these models to increase the yield of true positives and reduce the false-negative rate.[24]

DIFFICULTY IN APPROVAL BY THE CENTERS FOR MEDICARE & MEDICAID SERVICES

Despite the substantial associated survival benefit of LDCT demonstrated by the NLST, routine screening of high-risk patients with LDCT has not been widely adopted. In 2014, after reviewing the efficacy of LDCT, sputum cytology, and CXR in asymptomatic persons with average or high risk of developing lung cancer, the USPSTF updated their 2004 lung cancer screening recommendations

to call for annual LDCT screening examinations in high-risk patients. The USPSTF recommendations are targeted at asymptomatic adults aged 55 to 80 years who have a smoking history of at least 30 pack-years and currently smoke or have quit within the previous 15 years. Screening examinations are to be discontinued for any 1 of the following 3 reasons: (1) if a person reaches 15 years of not smoking, (2) if a patient develops a severe health problem limiting life expectancy, or (3) if a patient is either unwilling or medically unable to undergo lung surgery with curative intent. The USPSTF has designated these recommendations grade B, which suggests that providers offer this service, because it implies a high certainty that the net benefit is moderate. **Table 4** lists the current screening guidelines of the leading professional organizations—all of them largely follow the NLST criteria.[25]

Several studies have examined the NLST data from perspectives relevant for implementation. Stratification of the NLST patients into quintiles, as Bach and Gould have performed,[16] produces 3 intriguing perspectives. First, the number of participants needed to be screened to prevent 1 lung cancer death—therefore, a measure of benefit to a patient—varies from 161 for the highest risk to 5276 for the lowest risk, a 33-fold difference. Second, a measure of benefit-harm tradeoff in the form of false-positive results per prevented lung cancer death also varies dramatically (25-fold), from 1648 to 65 false-positive results per prevented death. Furthermore, de Koning and colleagues[26] have compiled modeling evidence based on NLST and Prostate, Lung, Colorectal and Ovarian Cancer Screening Trial data and suggest that approximately 50% of lung cancers can be detected at early stages if certain high-risk patients are screened annually. Based on their analysis, this would result in a 14% reduction in lung cancer mortality, translating to an estimated 521 lung cancer deaths prevented per 100,000 persons in the population. Additional subgroup analysis of NLST data also suggests that statistically significant reductions in mortality could be achieved for patients with adenocarcinoma (relative risk 0.75 [95% CI, 0.60 to 0.94]) but not for patients with other lung cancer histologic profiles.[27] Borderline statistically significant differences were also shown between men and women (relative risk 0.73 for women vs 0.92 for men; $P = .08$). In addition to the detection of 50% of cancers at early stages, 575 screening examinations per lung cancer death can be averted, with 5250 life-years gained per 100,000-member cohort. These modeling data are what prompted the USPSTF to broaden their target population

Table 4
Recommendations for lung cancer screening

Organization	Specified Population	Screening Recommendation	Comments
USPSTF[38]	• Age 55–80 • Minimum 30 pack-year smoking history • Current or former smoker within past 15 y	Annual LDCT	Grade B recommendation
American Cancer Society[40]	• Age 55–74 • Minimum 30 pack-year smoking history • Current or former smoker within past 15 y	Annual LDCT at experienced screening center Recommend against CXR	Discussion with patient before screening regarding harms and benefits
National Comprehensive Cancer Network Guidelines[41]	• Age 55–74 • Minimum 30 pack-year smoking history • Current or former smoker within past 15 y	Annual LDCT	Also recommend annual screening for those aged 50 and older with ≥20 pack-year smoking history, with additional comorbidity, with at least 5% risk of developing lung cancer during the next 5 y
American Association for Thoracic Surgery[42]	• Age 55–79 • Minimum 30 pack-year smoking history • Current or former smoker within past 15 y	Annual LDCT	Also recommend annual screening for those aged 50 and older with ≥20 pack-year smoking history, with additional comorbidity, with at least 5% risk of developing lung cancer during the next 5 y
American College of Chest Physicians, American Society of Clinical Oncology, American Thoracic Society[17]	• Age 55–74 • Minimum 30 pack-year smoking history • Current or former smoker within past 15 y	Annual LDCT	Screening settings should reflect NLST methods

Data from Humphrey L, Deffebach M, Pappas M, et al. U.S. Preventive Services Task Force Evidence Syntheses, formerly Systematic Evidence Reviews. In: Screening for lung cancer: systematic review to update the U.S. Preventive Services Task Force Recommendation. Rockville (MD): Agency for Healthcare Research and Quality (US); 2013.

beyond the population set out in the NLST to an upper age limit of 80 years and to recommend a maximum length of screening of 26 years as opposed to the 3 years of screening in the NLST protocol.[28] Such a screening program would not be without its harms, however, which are predicted to include 67,550 false-positive test results, 910 biopsies or surgeries for benign lesions, and 190 overdiagnosed cases of cancer. These potential harms, perhaps not surprisingly, play a central role in impeding the progress of broad implementation.[29]

A 2008 law, titled "Medicare Improvements for Patients and Providers Act," allows for the CMS to add new preventative services with USPSTF grade A or B recommendations, although it does not make doing so a requirement. Under the Patient Protection and Affordable Care Act of 2010, USPSTF grade A or B recommendations earn waivers for deductibles and copayments in private insurance and Medicare. These new A or B recommendations may also be applied to private health plans on an annual basis, according to the US Department of Health and Human Services.[29] Critically, for lung cancer screening, Medicare is not subject to the same mandate.[28] In April 2014, during the process of applying for CMS approval of LDCT screening, the Medicare Evidence

Development & Coverage Advisory Committee delivered a vote of low confidence that the benefits of LDCT would outweigh the harms among Medicare beneficiaries in a community setting. This ruling surprised many, given the promising results of the well-designed NLST and the grade B recommendation from the USPSTF.

Relevant to the decision of the CMS, however, is further analysis of the data that reveals more nuance in the context of the Medicare patient population. Only 25% of patients studied in the NLST were older than 65, fewer than 10% were 70 years or older, and none was over the age of 74.[28] Moreover, the potential harms associated with screening and its resulting work-ups are magnified in this population: older patients have higher complication rates from biopsy of pulmonary nodules,[30] have higher postoperative mortality when their disease is resected,[31] and are generally more susceptible to the harms of overtesting and overtreatment.[17] Other important considerations for CMS include diminishing returns of screening among an aging population and, perhaps most importantly, the costs associated with screening.

In the wake of the publication of the NLST in 2012, Goulart and colleagues[32] performed an economic analysis of the results. They found that LDCT screening will add $1.3 billion (in 2011 US dollars) in annual national health care expenditures, for an uptake rate of 50%, progressing to $2.0 billion, for an uptake rate of 75%. At a 75% screening rate, LDCT screening is expected to prevent 8100 premature lung cancer deaths, with the cost of screening to avoid 1 lung cancer death $240,000. Further economic analysis, this time in the form of an actuarial review, conducted by Pyenson and colleagues[33] (also in 2012), framed the discussion with relation to insurance coverage and reimbursement of LDCT screening. They found that the cost of lung cancer screening depends on various factors ranging from the number of people screened to the prices charged, types of screening, and screening quality. The investigators estimated the average annual cost of lung cancer screening to be $247 per person screened, assuming that 75% of the screenings are repeat procedures, which they reported as consistent with previous large-scale screening programs.[11] They developed 3 LDCT scenarios for cost per life-year saved, ranging from $11,708 to $26,016 (in 2012 US dollars) for lung cancer screening to $31,309 to $51,274 for breast cancer screening by mammography; $18,705 to $28,958 for colorectal cancer screening by colonoscopy; and $50,162 to $75,181 for cervical cancer screening by Papanicolaou smear. Their LDCT screening population was a high-risk population, in the United States,

aged 50 to 64 years, with a smoking history of at least 30 pack-years—a population that does not match the NLST participants in terms of age or align with the USPSTF recommendations. Nonetheless, their findings showed that screening would cost approximately $1 per insured member per month. The investigators also qualify their findings by instructing payers and patients to seek screening from high-quality, low-cost providers, which again poses necessary questions for any potential systems-based screening mechanism. Building on this study, Villanti and colleagues[34] added in the variables of quality-adjusted life-years (QALYs) to an analysis investigating the effects of smoking cessation, also using the same study population of a hypothetical cohort of 18 million adults between the ages of 50 and 64 with a smoking history of at least 30 pack-years. They reported a cost of $27.8 billion over 15 years, yielding 985,284 QALYs gained, for a cost-utility ratio of $28,240 per QALY gained (all in 2012 US dollars). Furthermore, they found that adding smoking cessation increased both the costs and the QALYs saved, with a range of cost-utility ratio from $16,198 per QALY gained to $23,185 per QALY gained. According to the investigators, these estimates show screening highly cost effective in their hypothetical high-risk cohort, especially when they include smoking cessation, which improved the cost-effectiveness of lung cancer screening by 20% to 45%.

Just as cost is an important practical consideration, patient adherence must also be thoroughly considered for any implementation of a screening program. Adherence to LDCT screening in the NLST was an uncharacteristically high 95%. The lessons from colon cancer screening show that follow-up is difficult in patients at the highest risk of developing disease.[35] Furthermore, studies have shown that smokers at a higher risk of developing lung cancer are less interested in being screened, even though they recognize their level of risk.[36] These concerns are also relevant when discussing implementation on a population-based level.

Accordingly, the USPSTF advocates for organized screening programs that include smoking cessation counseling when applicable, standardized scanning and image interpretation, quality standardization, and registry participation and validation to ensure that LDCT screening achieves results similar to those of the NLST.[37–39] Despite the NLST data, the myriad follow-up studies and analyses, and the favorable USPSTF recommendation, the prospect of broadly implementing LDCT screening for lung cancer in the United States will remain in doubt unless it is approved by the CMS.

SUMMARY

Screening protocols have become integrated as a standard of care for several solid tumor malignancies, including colon, prostate, and breast cancer. After the finding in the 2011 NLST of a 20% decrease in lung cancer–specific mortality when LDCT screening is performed in high-risk patients, screening recommendations have been brought forth by several leading organizations. Because of concerns about the cost and potential complications associated with false-positive screens, however, particularly in the elderly population, approval for LDCT lung cancer screening by CMS is lacking. As a result, the future of lung cancer screening remains elusive in the current political and social climate. Following the completion and submission of this article, the Centers for Medicare & Medicaid Services approved screening for lung cancer in selected, high-risk individuals. Many of the issues surrounding LDCT for lung cancer highlighted in this article remain relevant and will require continued investigation.

REFERENCES

1. Wender RC, Smith R, Harper D. Cancer screening. Prim Care 2002;29(3):697–725.
2. Siegel R, Ma J, Zou Z, et al. Cancer statistics, 2014. CA Cancer J Clin 2014;64(1):9–29.
3. Moyer VA. Screening for prostate cancer: U.S. Preventive Services Task Force recommendation statement. Ann Intern Med 2012;157(2):120–34.
4. DeSantis CE, Lin CC, Mariotto AB, et al. Cancer treatment and survivorship statistics, 2014. CA Cancer J Clin 2014;64(4):252–71.
5. Weinberg DS, Schoen RE. Screening for colorectal cancer. Ann Intern Med 2014;160(9).
6. Oken MM, Hocking WG, Kvale PA, et al. Screening by chest radiograph and lung cancer mortality: the Prostate, Lung, Colorectal, and Ovarian (PLCO) randomized trial. JAMA 2011;306(17):1865–73.
7. Berlin NI. Overview of the NCI cooperative early lung cancer detection program. Cancer 2000;89(11 Suppl):2349–51.
8. Melamed MR, Flehinger BJ, Zaman MB, et al. Screening for early lung cancer. Results of the Memorial Sloan-Kettering study in New York. Chest 1984;86(1):44–53.
9. Fontana RS, Sanderson DR, Woolner LB, et al. Lung cancer screening: the Mayo program. J Occup Med 1986;28(8):746–50.
10. Henschke CI, McCauley DI, Yankelevitz DF, et al. Early lung cancer action project: overall design and findings from baseline screening. Lancet 1999;354(9173):99–105.
11. Henschke CI, Yankelevitz DF, Libby DM, et al. Survival of patients with stage I lung cancer detected on CT screening. N Engl J Med 2006; 355(17):1763–71.
12. Pastorino U, Bellomi M, Landoni C, et al. Early lung-cancer detection with spiral CT and positron emission tomography in heavy smokers: 2-year results. Lancet 2003;362(9384):593–7.
13. Swensen SJ, Jett JR, Hartman TE, et al. Lung cancer screening with CT: Mayo Clinic experience. Radiology 2003;226(3):756–61.
14. Aberle DR, Adams AM, Berg CD, et al. Reduced lung-cancer mortality with low-dose computed tomographic screening. N Engl J Med 2011; 365(5):395–409.
15. Aberle DR, Berg CD, Black WC, et al. The national lung screening trial: overview and study design. Radiology 2011;258(1):243–53.
16. Bach PB, Gould MK. When the average applies to no one: personalized decision making about potential benefits of lung cancer screening. Ann Intern Med 2012;157(8):571–3.
17. Bach PB, Mirkin JN, Oliver TK, et al. Benefits and harms of CT screening for lung cancer: a systematic review. JAMA 2012;307(22):2418–29.
18. Aberle DR, DeMello S, Berg CD, et al. Results of the two incidence screenings in the national lung screening trial. N Engl J Med 2013;369(10):920–31.
19. Church TR, Black WC, Aberle DR, et al. Results of initial low-dose computed tomographic screening for lung cancer. N Engl J Med 2013;368(21):1980–91.
20. Pace LE, Keating NL. A systematic assessment of benefits and risks to guide breast cancer screening decisions. JAMA 2014;311(13):1327–35.
21. Bleyer A, Welch HG. Effect of three decades of screening mammography on breast-cancer incidence. N Engl J Med 2012;367(21):1998–2005.
22. Brenner DJ. Radiation risks potentially associated with low-dose CT screening of adult smokers for lung cancer. Radiology 2004;231(2):440–5.
23. Brenner DJ, Hall EJ. Computed tomography–an increasing source of radiation exposure. N Engl J Med 2007;357(22):2277–84.
24. Brawley OW, Flenaugh EL. Low-dose spiral CT screening and evaluation of the solitary pulmonary nodule. Oncology (Williston Park) 2014;28(5):441–6.
25. Humphrey L, Deffebach M, Pappas M, et al. Screening for Lung Cancer: Systematic Review to Update the U.S. Preventive Services Task Force Recommendation. Evidence Synthesis No. 105. AHRQ Publication No. 13-05188-EF-1. Rockville (MD): Agency for Healthcare Research and Quality; 2013. Available at: http://www.ncbi.nlm.nih.gov/pubmedhealth/PMH0060145/.
26. de Koning HJ, Meza R, Plevritis SK, et al. Benefits and harms of computed tomography lung cancer screening strategies: a comparative modeling study

for the U.S. Preventive Services Task Force. Ann Intern Med 2014;160(5):311–20.

27. Pinsky PF, Church TR, Izmirlian G, et al. The national lung screening trial: results stratified by demographics, smoking history, and lung cancer histology. Cancer 2013;119(22):3976–83.

28. Bach PB. Raising the bar for the U.S. Preventive Services Task Force. Ann Intern Med 2014;160(5): 365–6.

29. Wiener RS. Balancing the benefits and harms of low-dose computed tomography screening for lung cancer: medicare's options for coverage. Ann Intern Med 2014;161(6):445–6.

30. Wiener RS, Schwartz LM, Woloshin S, et al. Population-based risk for complications after transthoracic needle lung biopsy of a pulmonary nodule: an analysis of discharge records. Ann Intern Med 2011; 155(3):137–44.

31. Kozower BD, Sheng S, O'Brien SM, et al. STS database risk models: predictors of mortality and major morbidity for lung cancer resection. Ann Thorac Surg 2010;90(3):875–81 [discussion: 881–3].

32. Goulart BH, Bensink ME, Mummy DG, et al. Lung cancer screening with low-dose computed tomography: costs, national expenditures, and cost-effectiveness. J Natl Compr Canc Netw 2012; 10(2):267–75.

33. Pyenson BS, Sander MS, Jiang Y, et al. An actuarial analysis shows that offering lung cancer screening as an insurance benefit would save lives at relatively low cost. Health Aff (Millwood) 2012;31(4):770–9.

34. Villanti AC, Jiang Y, Abrams DB, et al. A cost-utility analysis of lung cancer screening and the additional benefits of incorporating smoking cessation interventions. PLoS One 2013;8(8):e71379.

35. Baig N, Myers RE, Turner BJ, et al. Physician-reported reasons for limited follow-up of patients with a positive fecal occult blood test screening result. Am J Gastroenterol 2003;98(9):2078–81.

36. Silvestri GA, Nietert PJ, Zoller J, et al. Attitudes towards screening for lung cancer among smokers and their non-smoking counterparts. Thorax 2007; 62(2):126–30.

37. Detterbeck FC, Unger M. Screening for lung cancer: moving into a new era. Ann Intern Med 2014;160(5): 363–4.

38. Moyer VA. Screening for lung cancer: U.S. Preventive Services Task Force recommendation statement. Ann Intern Med 2014;160(5):330–8.

39. Recommendations. U.S. Preventive Services Task Force. 2014. Available at: http://www.uspreventiveservicestaskforce.org/recommendations.htm. Accessed July 30, 2014.

40. Wender R, Fontham ET, Barrera E Jr, et al. American Cancer Society lung cancer screening guidelines. CA Cancer J Clin 2013;63(2):107–17.

41. National Comprehensive Cancer Center. NCCN Clinical Practice Guidelines in oncology: lung cancer screening. Available at: http://www.nccn.org/professionals/physician_gls/pdf/lung_screening.pdf. Accessed July 30, 2014.

42. Jaklitsch MT, Jacobson FL, Austin JH, et al. The American Association for Thoracic Surgery guidelines for lung cancer screening using low-dose computed tomography scans for lung cancer survivors and other high-risk groups. J Thorac Cardiovasc Surg 2012;144(1):33–8.

Health Risks from Computed Tomographic Screening

Seth B. Krantz, MD[a],*, Bryan F. Meyers, MD[b]

KEYWORDS

- Lung cancer • Screening • Risks • Overdiagnosis

KEY POINTS

- Low-dose computed tomographic (CT) (LDCT) scan screening of patients at increased risk for lung cancer has shown a survival benefit but is not without risk.
- Although the radiation dose is low, screening often leads to additional higher-dose studies, which cumulatively increase the radiation exposure and provide a measurable increase in cancer risk.
- The false-positive rate from screening is not insignificant and can lead to additional diagnostic procedures for what is ultimately determined to be benign disease. These procedures have their own inherent complication rate.
- Overdiagnosis leads to the treatment of cancers that would otherwise be clinically insignificant, which means unhelpful major surgery, radiation therapy, and chemotherapy for indolent cancers that would not have otherwise affected the patient's survival or quality of life.

INTRODUCTION

Based largely on the results of the National Lung Screening Trial (NLST),[1] the US Preventive Services Task Force (USPSTF)[2] now recommends screening for lung cancer with LDCT for high-risk patients. The benefits, although significant, must be balanced against the risk inherent to any intervention, including screening. Unlike the risks of new medications or procedures, the potential harms from noninvasive screening tests are harder to see and often overlooked. The primary risks for lung cancer screening with CT are radiation exposure, false-positive results with the resulting invasive diagnostic procedures, overdiagnosis and overtreatment of indolent or nonlethal cancers, and the paradoxic encouragement of high-risk behavior, that is, smoking, in patients with

negative screen results. These risks have the potential to undermine the mortality benefit achieved with screening and are a critical aspect of the discussion that must occur with patients considering enrollment in a screening program.

DIRECT HARM FROM SCREENING: RADIATION EXPOSURE

Although often seen as benign and noninvasive, radiographic screening does pose a direct risk to the patient in the form of radiation exposure. With the increasing use of CT scanning across medical practice, there has been renewed interest in studying the potential harm from cumulative radiation exposure. The actual risk of low-dose radiation exposure from medical imaging and procedures remains uncertain. Most of the data

Disclosures: None.
[a] Division of Cardiothoracic Surgery, Department of Surgery, Washington University School of Medicine, 660 South Euclid Avenue, Campus Box: 8234, St Louis, MO 63110, USA; [b] Section of Thoracic Surgery, Division of Cardiothoracic Surgery, Department of Surgery, Washington University School of Medicine, 660 South Euclid Avenue, Campus Box: 8234, St Louis, MO 63110, USA
* Corresponding author.
E-mail address: krantzs@wudosis.wustl.edu

Thorac Surg Clin 25 (2015) 155–160
http://dx.doi.org/10.1016/j.thorsurg.2014.11.003

on low-dose radiation exposure comes from either nuclear power workers or survivors of atomic bombs.[3] Standardization of radiation exposure into Sievert units, which takes into account the different effects various types of ionizing radiation have on tissues, allows some comparison and clinically useful extrapolation to the exposures seen with medical imaging.

Patients in the NLST received several annual LDCT scans, each with an average of 1.5 mSv, which represents a significantly lower radiation dose than the high-resolution CT used for typical diagnostic indications.[3] However, the cumulative dose for a typical patient, screened from age 50 years to age 74 years, is thus in the 30-mSv range, which is associated with increased cancer risk. A 15-country analysis of more than 400,000 nuclear power workers found a significant dose-dependent increase in all-cause mortality and cancer-specific mortality. The primary risk of cancer death was from lung cancer.[4] In a large cohort study of more than 85,000 atomic bomb survivors, excess cancer risk exists for estimated exposure doses as low as 5 mSv.[5] The estimated risk of developing lung cancer directly related to the radiation from screening has been reported up to 0.85% over the course of a 25-year screening program. Extrapolated to population-based screening of high-risk patients, this would represent a 1.8% increase in new lung cancers, which would reduce, but not eliminate, the mortality benefit from screening the high-risk patients for whom screening is indicated.[6]

Most epidemiologic studies of cancer risk related to medical radiation exposure have been performed in children. These results may not reflect the same risks as in adults aged 50 years or higher undergoing screening, as children and younger adults have a much longer time horizon for the DNA changes from ionizing radiation to develop into malignancies. A study modeling risk of cancer from surveillance CT scan in patients undergoing endovascular aortic repair for aortic aneurysm and dissection showed a significant risk reduction by limiting scans to once every 3 or 5 years, as compared with the risk seen with standard yearly surveillance. In their model, the effective relative risk (ERR) of cancer decreased with decreasing age. Patients aged 50 to 55 years, the earliest age of entry in the NLST, showed the highest ERR for the development of new cancers.[7] Doses used in their model were 15 mSv for non-contrast CT and 31 mSv for contrast CT, which are significantly higher than those for low-dose chest CT used for lung cancer screening (1.5 mSv).

The overall risk from low-dose radiation from medical imaging remains a point of significant controversy. The above-mentioned studies refer to what is known as the linear no-threshold model, in which there is no threshold dose for harm, the risk is linear, and the risk at low doses can be determined from the available data on the risk at higher doses.[3] There is some evidence that this may not be accurate and in some cases actually underestimate the risk of LDCT.[8] True epidemiologic studies of very low-dose radiation remain limited. The American Association of Physicists in Medicine in their official policy statement, claim the following:

> Risks of medical imaging at effective doses below 50 mSv for single procedures or 100 mSv for multiple procedures over short time periods are too low to be detectable and may be nonexistent. Predictions of hypothetical cancer incidence and deaths in patient populations exposed to such low doses are highly speculative and should be discouraged.

Screening LDCT scanning, as discussed later, frequently leads to additional diagnostic studies, either traditional thin-slice, high-resolution CT or PET-CT, with higher effective radiation doses than screening studies. Thus, the true level of exposure due to a screening program is more than simply the cumulative effect of the LDCT. The best available data suggest a real and measurable risk that must be accounted for when measuring the mortality benefit associated with screening. The magnitude of that risk may take decades to become truly evident.

Risks Posed by False-Positive Screen Results

Unlike the small potential risk from radiation exposure, the harm from false-positive results of screening tests is more pervasive yet harder for patients and physicians alike to appreciate. With cancer screening, false-positive screening test results frequently lead to invasive procedures to obtain a definitive tissue diagnosis. Much has been published with respect to the implications of false-positive screen outcomes, primarily with breast and prostate cancer, which have a much longer screening history from which to draw data. With prostate cancer screening with the serologic biomarker prostate specific antigen (PSA), the false-positive rate for a PSA value cutoff of 2.5 to 4 can be as high as 80% with a 10-year biopsy rate of 10%.[9] Up to a third of those patients complain of a significant adverse effect from the biopsy.[10] In breast cancer screening using annual mammography, the false-positive rate can be as high as 50% per patient after 10 screening mammograms. For every breast cancer case that is diagnosed, this means 47 women have required additional imaging studies and 5 women have undergone invasive procedures.[11]

Data specific to the burden of false-positive results in lung cancer screening is limited to the recent randomized and cohort trials that sought to validate the role of screening. Although the number of patients in these trials is small in comparison to the number of patients who have undergone screening for breast and prostate cancer in actual clinical practice over the past several decades, it provides some sobering information about potential harms of screening. A meta-analysis of 8 randomized trials and 13 cohort studies found the average new nodule detection rate per round of screening to be 20%, yet more than 90% of the new nodules detected were benign.[12] In the NLST, the new detection rate was as high as 28% in the second round of screening and fell to 17% only at the third round, with 98% and 95% of those nodules being benign, respectively.[1] The proper handling of false-positive results is important in minimizing harm from such screening practices.

Raw false-positivity rate in screening, although important, is a crude measure. Screening, by definition, seeks to maximize sensitivity (finding the condition in the at-risk population) with specificity (distinguishing disease from false-positive results) typically obtained from further testing. This further testing has measurable costs to both the patient and the society (**Table 1**). The percentage of patients in the NLST who underwent additional CT imaging was 33%, and the number of patients who underwent PET was approximately 5%, which was fairly consistent across several randomized controlled trials and cohort studies.[12] With respect to noninvasive and invasive procedures, 1.2% of patients screened underwent noninvasive procedures (eg, bronchoscopy,

transthoracic needle biopsy) for what was shown to be benign disease. Half as many (0.6% of patients screened) underwent invasive excisional biopsy for what was ultimately shown to be a benign nodule. Of those patients who had a noninvasive procedure, 73% were benign. Clinicians in the trial were much more selective about who received an invasive surgical procedure, but despite that selectivity, 24% of all patients undergoing an invasive surgical biopsy had benign disease. Given the small number of patients who underwent invasive procedures, the overall risk of major complication was low; 0.045% in patients who did not have cancer compared with 0.33% for the entire screened population.[12] Among those patients who underwent invasive procedures, the complication rate was higher in those with lung cancer than in those with benign disease. Still among those patients who did not have lung cancer, the complication rate was 16% after surgical biopsy and more than 10% after needle biopsy. For needle biopsy, nearly all complications were classified as intermediate in severity.[1]

There is also a psychological risk to screening, in that 90% to 95% of the positive results in the initial screens will eventually be shown to be false-positive results. The burden of harboring a suspicious lung lesion is real, and the anxiety that results in the screened patient is clinically observable. A meta-analysis specifically studying patient-centered outcomes showed a short-term increase in distress in patients who had a false-positive screen result, although their distress levels returned to baseline at 2-year follow-up.[13] The overall weight of this complication of screening is currently unmeasurable.

Overdiagnosis

Perhaps even more difficult to appreciate than false positivity is the notion of overdiagnosis and overtreatment of indolent cancers, which has been a significant concern in both breast and prostate cancer, with estimates of overdiagnosis rates of 25% and 67%, respectively, and the concept has been a driving force in the changing recommendations from the USPSTF.[9,11,14] Determining the overdiagnosis rate requires knowledge of how many excess cancers are found by a screening trial and long-term outcomes data to determine what fraction of those cancers would have been clinically significant. For chest radiography and sputum lung cancer screening, the overdiagnosis rate was estimated to be 50%.[14,15] These investigators determined the number of overdiagnosed cancers by first determining the number of additional cancers found via a screening program compared with unscreened

---

Table 1
Of patients who had further diagnostic testing, percentage that underwent the various diagnostic modalities

Variable	Low-Dose CT (%)
Further imaging	57.9
Bronchoscopy	3.8
Percutaneous biopsy	3.5
Surgical procedure	4

Data from National Lung Screening Trial Research Team, Aberle DR, Adams AM, et al. Reduced lung-cancer mortality with low-dose computed tomographic screening. N Engl J Med 2011;365(5):395–409.

patients. On long-term follow-up, unscreened patients developed more new cancers than screened patients; these "catch-up" cancers represent cancers that became clinically apparent with time and thus would have benefited from being found at screening. The remaining excess represented the number of overdiagnosed cancers (**Fig. 1**). Similar methodology was applied to the NLST, and a potential overdiagnosis rate of 18% was shown in the LDCT group.[16] In the NLST, after the completion of screening, the difference between the 2 groups was 370 cancers (649 vs 279). During the 6 years of follow-up, there were 250 catch-up cancers, with a remaining difference narrowed to 120 cancers (1089 in the LDCT and 969 in the radiography arm), with this difference representing the estimated number of overdiagnosed cancers. There was significant variation in the rate of overdiagnosis depending on the tumor histology. For non–small cell lung cancer (NSCLC) the rate was 22.5%, whereas the rate for noninvasive adenocarcinoma (formerly bronchioaveolar carcinoma (BAC)) was 78.9% (**Table 2**). The investigators of this study also applied a statistical model to the data in an attempt to find a true actuarial overdiagnosis rate beyond the limited 6-year follow-up in the NLST. Using that model, overdiagnosis rates decrease as more slow-growing tumors would become clinically significant with increased follow-up. Overdiagnosis rates were 9% for all NSCLC, 1.2% for invasive NSLC, and 41% for noninvasive adenocarcinoma (BAC).[16]

Some of the challenge with overdiagnosis is the heterogeneity of tumor growth. Even with a generally aggressive cancer, such as NSCLC, tumors show a wide range of growth patterns. One single-center retrospective review of a prospectively screened cohort estimated that up to 25% of incident tumors were slow growing or indolent. In this

Table 2
Estimated overdiagnosis rates based on data from the NLST

Cancer Type	Overdiagnosis (%)
All lung cancers	18.5
All NSCLC, including BAC	22.5
All NSCLC, excluding BAC	11.7
BAC only	78.0

Data from Patz EF, Pinsky P, Gatsonis C, et al. Overdiagnosis in low-dose computed tomography screening for lung cancer. JAMA Intern Med 2014;174:269–74. http://dx.doi.org/10.1001/jamainternmed.2013.12738; and National Lung Screening Trial Research Team, Aberle DR, Adams AM, et al. Reduced lung-cancer mortality with low-dose computed tomographic screening. N Engl J Med 2011;365(5):395–409.

study, 18 of 120 (15%) new cancers diagnosed from previously imaged nodules showed a doubling time between 400 and 600 days (slow growing) and 13 of 120 (11%) showed a doubling time greater than 600 days (indolent).[17] The lung cancer–specific mortality in these patients with slow and indolent tumors was low, 0.9% per year, compared with 9.2% per year for patients with newly diagnosed cancers that were not present as nodules on prior screening. Patients with fast-growing cancers, diagnosed from previously seen nodules, had an annual mortality of 4.1%, although this difference was not statistically significant compared with slow-growing and indolent tumors.[17]

SMOKING BEHAVIOR

A theoretic risk of screening is that the 80% of screened patients with a negative screen lose some incentive to quit and it may in fact encourage

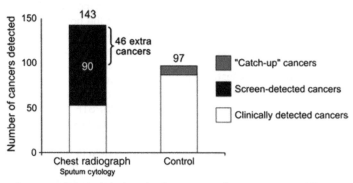

Fig. 1. Total number of cancers detected during the 6-year screening program and 5 years of additional follow-up. The catch-up cancers in the control group represent cancers that became clinically apparent during the follow-up period and thus presumably would have been found earlier with a screening program. The remaining extra cancers after accounting for these catch-up cancers represent the overdiagnosed cancers in the screening group. (*From* Welch HG, Black WC. Overdiagnosis in cancer. J Natl Cancer Inst 2010;102:608. http://dx.doi.org/10.1093/jnci/djq099; with permission.)

them to continue smoking. Analysis from the Dutch lung cancer screening program has shown that in general this is not the case. Patients enrolled in the screening trial overall showed a higher cessation rate than the general population. The control group had a higher quit rate, but this was not significant on intention to treat analysis.[18] Although there was no difference in quit rates between control groups and screened groups, patients in the screen group who had findings that required follow-up imaging were more likely to quit than patients with normal findings on screening CT.[19] It is uncertain whether the so-called teachable moment that occurs with a positive screen result is counterbalanced by the tacit encouragement to smoke that comes from a clearly negative screen result.

SUMMARY

Whether or not to recommend any medical treatment depends on weighing the benefits versus risks and on the level of evidence for each. The NLST provided good evidence on the overall survival benefit for a LDCT-based screening program on patients at high risk for developing lung cancer. Without large numbers of patients and extended follow-up, the risks of screening are more difficult to measure and were thus less clear from the NLST. Even the manner in which risks are classified is poorly defined, and a better framework for describing and studying the risks of screening may improve data.[20] Regardless, the primary risks remain radiation exposure, false-positive results with associated unnecessary imaging and additional procedures with their own inherent risk, and, perhaps most significantly, overdiagnosis. Overdiagnosis not merely exposes patients to small increased doses of radiation from further imaging or minimally invasive diagnostic procedures but also allows unhelpful major surgery, therapeutic radiation, and chemotherapy. Based on the data available from the NLST and Prostate, Lung, Colorectal, and Ovarian Cancer Screening Trial (PLCO), a modeling study for the USPSTF of more than 500 different screening programs was performed for a hypothetical 100,000 patient cohort of the general population.[21] In this analysis, 19,300 individuals would be eligible for screening. The optimal screening program closely followed the NLST criteria, with annual LDCT from age 55 years through age 80 years. Under this program, there would be 67,000 false-positive results (3.5 false-positive results per patient screened), 910 biopsies of benign lesions, and 190 overdiagnosed cancers, which was 3.7% of all estimated diagnosed lung cancers in this model; this was

balanced against 10.6 life-years gained per patient for each cancer diagnosed, a 14% reduction in lung cancer mortality for the entire cohort, and a 25% reduction in lung cancer mortality for screen-eligible patients. Overall risk benefit in this model favored implantation of a screening program, and USPSTF has recommended screening based on the NLST protocol. Screening is a potentially powerful tool in the fight to reduce morbidity and mortality from lung cancer; however, like any intervention, screening has real risks. To have maximum benefit for patients, these risks must be adequately documented and appropriately managed.

REFERENCES

1. National Lung Screening Trial Research Team, Aberle DR, Adams AM, et al. Reduced lung-cancer mortality with low-dose computed tomographic screening. N Engl J Med 2011;365:395–409. http://dx.doi.org/10.1056/NEJMoa1102873.
2. Humphrey LL, Deffebach M, Pappas M, et al. Screening for lung cancer with low-dose computed tomography: a systematic review to update the US Preventive Services Task Force recommendation. Ann Intern Med 2013;159:411–20. http://dx.doi.org/10.7326/0003-4819-159-6-201309170-00690.
3. Albert JM. Radiation risk from CT: implications for cancer screening. AJR Am J Roentgenol 2013;201: W81–7. http://dx.doi.org/10.2214/AJR.12.9226.
4. Cardis E, Vrijheid M, Blettner M, et al. The 15-Country Collaborative Study of Cancer Risk among Radiation Workers in the Nuclear Industry: estimates of radiation-related cancer risks. Radiat Res 2007; 167:396–416. http://dx.doi.org/10.1667/RR0553.1.
5. Preston DL, Pierce DA, Shimizu Y. Age-time patterns for cancer and noncancer excess risks in the atomic bomb survivors. Radiat Res 2000;154:733–4 [discussion: 734–5].
6. Brenner DJ. Radiation risks potentially associated with low-dose CT screening of adult smokers for lung cancer. Radiology 2004;231:440–5.
7. Motaganahalli R, Martin A, Feliciano B, et al. Estimating the risk of solid organ malignancy in patients undergoing routine computed tomography scans after endovascular aneurysm repair. J Vasc Surg 2012;56:929–37. http://dx.doi.org/10.1016/j.jvs.2012.02.061.
8. Brenner DJ, Doll R, Goodhead DT, et al. Cancer risks attributable to low doses of ionizing radiation: assessing what we really know. Proc Natl Acad Sci U S A 2003;100:13761–6.
9. Moyer VA. Screening for prostate cancer: U.S. Preventive Services Task Force recommendation statement. Ann Intern Med 2012;157:120–34. http://dx.doi.org/10.7326/0003-4819-157-2-201207170-00459.
10. Rosario DJ, Lane JA, Metcalfe C, et al. Short term outcomes of prostate biopsy in men tested for

cancer by prostate specific antigen: prospective evaluation within ProtecT study. BMJ 2012;344: d7894.

11. Nelson HD, Tyne K, Naik A, et al. Screening for breast cancer: an update for the U.S. Preventive Services Task Force. Ann Intern Med 2009;151: 727–37. http://dx.doi.org/10.7326/0003-4819-151-10-200911170-00009. W237–42.

12. Bach PB, Mirkin JN, Oliver TK, et al. Benefits and harms of CT screening for lung cancer: a systematic review. JAMA 2012;307:2418–29. http://dx.doi.org/10.1001/jama.2012.5521.

13. Slatore CG, Sullivan DR, Pappas M, et al. Patient-centered outcomes among lung cancer screening recipients with computed tomography: a systematic review. J Thorac Oncol 2014;9:927–34. http://dx.doi.org/10.1097/JTO.0000000000000210.

14. Welch HG, Black WC. Overdiagnosis in cancer. J Natl Cancer Inst 2010;102:605–13. http://dx.doi.org/10.1093/jnci/djq099.

15. Fontana RS, Sanderson DR, Woolner LB, et al. Screening for lung cancer. A critique of the Mayo Lung Project. Cancer 1991;67:1155–64.

16. Patz EF, Pinsky P, Gatsonis C, et al. Overdiagnosis in low-dose computed tomography screening for lung cancer. JAMA Intern Med 2014;174:269–74. http://dx.doi.org/10.1001/jamainternmed.2013.12738.

17. Veronesi G, Maisonneuve P, Bellomi M, et al. Estimating overdiagnosis in low-dose computed tomography screening for lung cancer: a cohort study. Ann Intern Med 2012;157:776–84. http://dx.doi.org/10.7326/0003-4819-157-11-201212040-00005.

18. van der Aalst CM, van den Bergh KA, Willemsen MC, et al. Lung cancer screening and smoking abstinence: 2 year follow-up data from the Dutch-Belgian randomised controlled lung cancer screening trial. Thorax 2010;65:600–5. http://dx.doi.org/10.1136/thx.2009.133751.

19. Ashraf H, Tonnesen P, Holst Pedersen J, et al. Effect of CT screening on smoking habits at 1-year follow-up in the Danish Lung Cancer Screening Trial (DLCST). Thorax 2009;64:388–92. http://dx.doi.org/10.1136/thx.2008.102475.

20. Harris RP, Sheridan SL, Lewis CL, et al. The harms of screening: a proposed taxonomy and application to lung cancer screening. JAMA Intern Med 2014;174: 281–5. http://dx.doi.org/10.1001/jamainternmed.2013.12745.

21. de Koning HJ, Meza R, Plevritis SK, et al. Benefits and harms of computed tomography lung cancer screening strategies: a comparative modeling study for the U.S. Preventive Services Task Force. Ann Intern Med 2014;160:311–20. http://dx.doi.org/10.7326/M13-2316.

Lung Cancer Screening
The European Perspective

Giulia Veronesi, MD

KEYWORDS

- Lung cancer • Early-stage lung cancer • Computed tomography • Diagnostic algorithm • Survival

KEY POINTS

- European studies have contributed significantly to understanding of lung cancer screening.
- Smoking within screening, quality of life, nodule management, minimally invasive treatments, cancer prevention programs, and risk models have been extensively investigated by European groups.
- Mortality data from European screening studies have not been encouraging so far, but long-term results of the NELSON study (The Dutch-Belgian Randomized Lung Cancer Screening Trial [Dutch acronym: NELSON study]) are eagerly awaited.
- Investigations on molecular markers of lung cancer are ongoing in Europe; preliminary results suggest they may become an important screening tool in the future.

INTRODUCTION: THE EXTENT OF THE PROBLEM

Lung cancer is a leading cause of death worldwide. Incidence continues to grow among women in developed countries and across the board in developing countries.[1] Single-arm and randomized studies on early lung cancer detection with low-dose computed tomography (LDCT) without contrast have shown that the technology is highly sensitive for detecting small lung nodules, with limited radiation exposure, acceptable costs, and short examination times.[2–5]

The large randomized National Lung Screening Trial (NLST), published in 2011, recruited 53,000 high-risk smoker volunteers over 55 years of age. It demonstrated a mortality reduction of 20% in the LDCT-screened group compared with the group screened by chest radiograph.[6] Previous nonrandomized studies had also estimated a mortality reduction of between 23% and 64% compared with historical control cohorts.[7,8] The National Cancer Comprehensive Network and US Preventive Services Task Force have recommended annual LDCT screening for lung cancer in high-risk individuals.[9,10]

The contributions of European investigators to lung cancer screening are mainly in the fields of primary prevention and chemoprevention associated with screening, risk assessment models, new algorithms for nodule management, and minimally invasive and conservative treatments for screening-detected nodules. European studies on molecular markers for the early detection of lung cancer are ongoing and have produced promising results.[11,12] Several European randomized studies were underpowered and failed to demonstrate that LDCT screening could reduce mortality, whereas the largest European randomized study—NELSON—has not yet released mortality data for the 2 study arms.

In Europe, approximately 269,000 deaths from lung cancer are expected in 2014 and it now seems clear that screening and early detection can contribute to reducing lung cancer mortality. Although antismoking campaigns are having an effect and must be continued, lung cancer screening has yet to be implemented on a large scale and remains a public health priority for Europe.[12]

PRIMARY PREVENTION AND CHEMOPREVENTION IN ASSOCIATION WITH SCREENING

Primary prevention remains a cornerstone of the fight against lung cancer. Cigarette smoking causes approximately 90% of lung cancers.[13]

The author has nothing to disclose.
Lung Cancer Early Detection Unit, European Institute of Oncology, Via Ripamonti 435, 20141 Milan, Italy
E-mail address: giulia.veronesi@ieo.it

The health benefits of stopping smoking cessation are well documented and extend well beyond reducing the risk of developing lung cancer.[14] Stopping smoking proves difficult for most people, however, and cannot be achieved without determination and without help in the form of specific smoking cessation programs.

Those interested in participating in screening for lung cancer (usually heavy smokers) have, by their willingness to participate, expressed a desire for better health. They are, therefore, likely to be receptive to smoking cessation programs, which should be implemented alongside lung cancer screening, as also urged by screening guidelines.[15]

Several European studies have investigated smoking behavior in the context of screening. The effect of screening on smoking was investigated over 1 year in those recruited to the randomized Danish Lung Cancer Screening Trial (DLCST).[16] It was found that screening did not actually favor smoking cessation, emphasizing the need for an effective additional intervention to encourage cessation. A positive scan result was highly stressful, however, and did favor smoking cessation. Finally, the study found that screening did not facilitate continuation of smoking, as has been claimed by detractors of screening.

By contrast, the smoking abstinence investigation part of the NELSON randomized study[17] did not find that a positive scan result had a positive effect on stopping smoking; however, the investigators agreed that presentation of the test outcome represented an excellent opportunity for encouraging smoking cessation. One objective of the NELSON study was to assess whether a tailored self-help intervention was more effective than a standard brochure in getting long-term male smokers to stop smoking.[18] It was found that tailored smoking cessation information had no advantage over standard self-help information after 2 years of follow-up. Only a low percentage of participants, however, actually received the tailored advice. This is important information for future screening program start-ups.

Another approach to prevention is to use chemopreventive agents to block the progression of precancerous lesions and promote lung tissue repair by mechanisms, such as suppression of inflammation and growth, restoration of normal epithelial differentiation, and improving immune surveillance. All methods tested in phase III chemoprevention studies have so far proved ineffective.[19] Screening programs offer ideal populations for testing potential chemopreventive agents using new intermediate endpoints, such as disappearance/reduction of peripheral lung nodules.

To assess the effect of budesonide—a potentially chemopreventive glucocorticoid—on CT-detected nodules, the author's group performed a randomized double-blind phase IIb trial of inhaled budesonide versus inhaled placebo in current and former smokers with CT-detected target lung nodules (that had persisted for at least a year but did not require additional diagnostic ascertainment according to the COSMOS [Continuous Observation of SMOking Subjects] protocol).[20] A total of 202 individuals received inhaled budesonide, 800 mg twice daily, or placebo for 1 year. The primary endpoint was the effect of budesonide on target nodule size in a per-person analysis after 1 year. Although the per-person analysis did not show a significant difference between the 2 arms, the per-lesion analysis revealed that budesonide was significantly ($P = .02$) associated with the regression of nonsolid target nodules (**Fig. 1**). The results were confirmed after 5 years: mean nonsolid nodule diameter significantly reduced in those who had received budesonide for a year compared with controls. This study, nested in the COSMOS screening study, revealed a new endpoint: peripheral ground-glass opacities on LDCT, which are likely to be atypical adenomatous hyperplasias or adenocarcinomas in situ. These lesions will be targeted in a future study using low-dose oral aspirin. Long-term aspirin use has been associated with reduced lung cancer mortality in large meta-analyses.[21,22]

NODULE MANAGEMENT

The frequent finding of indeterminate noncalcified lung nodules remains a problem with LDCT screening for lung cancer. To reduce the number of useless investigations and consequent risk of morbidity in screened subjects, standardized algorithms for managing indeterminate lung nodules have been developed to achieve a balance between a too invasive approach and a too lax approach that risks diagnosing the cancer at a later stage. Only if lung cancer is diagnosed early does it have a reasonable chance of being cured. Single-arm studies report that approximately 80% of screening-detected cases are detected at stage I or II[23,24]—compared with 16% at this stage in historical data on unscreened individuals[25]—and the resection rate is approximately 80% to 90%. **Fig. 2** summarizes Surveillance, Epidemiology, and End Results (SEER [Statistics and Epidemiology End Results]) population-based data on the stage distribution of lung cancers at diagnosis. **Fig. 2** also shows population-based relative survival (according to SEER summary stage) for lung cancer patients.

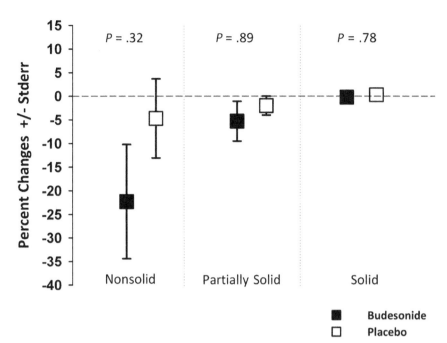

Fig. 1. Percent changes in maximum diameters of indeterminate lung nodules according to type of nodule by treatment arm (inhaled budesonide vs placebo for 1 year). (*From* Veronesi G, Szabo E, Decensi A, et al. Randomized phase II trial of inhaled budesonide vs placebo in high-risk individuals with CT screen-detected lung nodules. Cancer Prev Res (Phila) 2011;4:40; with permission.)

The size threshold for considering a nodule as positive varies greatly between screening studies.[23,24,26] A 2011 review[27] reported experience of North American and European screening trials: summary data for selected trials are shown in **Table 1**. Most trials reported high (19%–32%) proportions of total invasive procedures for what turned out to be benign disease and high proportions (16%–28%) of total volunteers recalled for further investigations.

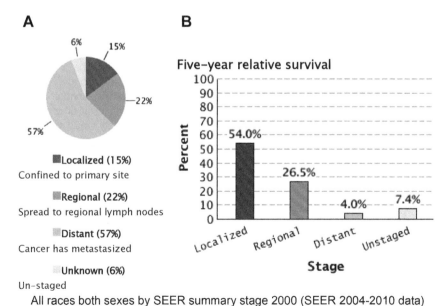

Fig. 2. Percentage of cases by stage at diagnosis and 5-year relative survival for cancers of lung and bronchus. (A) Graphic of stage distribution according to SEER data; (B) 5 years relative survival according to data from SEERS database. (*From* National Cancer Institute. Surveillance Epidemiology and End Results. National Institute of Health; 2013. Available at: http://seer.cancer.gov/statfacts/html/lungb.html. Accessed November 26, 2014.)

The largest European randomized trial, the NELSON study,[26] was the first to incorporate software-calculated volume doubling times (VDTs) of nodules into a management algorithm. Nodules less than 50 mm^3 (4.6 mm diameter) were considered negative; those greater than 500 mm^3 (>9.8 mm diameter) were positive; and those in the 50 to 500 mm^3 range were indeterminate; 21% of subjects (first round) had indeterminate nodules and were recalled for repeat LDCT at 3 months: VDTs were then used to direct these either to further investigation or just follow-up. Using this 2-step approach, only 2.6% of baseline NELSON scans were considered positive at baseline; however, approximately 27% of surgical patients underwent invasive procedure for a benign disease.

For the author's COSMOS single-arm trial, a noninvasive protocol for nodule work-up, involving routine use of positron emission tomography (PET)-CT and VDT, instead of CT-guided lung biopsy, was developed and refined.[23] **Table 2** summarizes 5 years of COSMOS data, showing low recall rates (10% at baseline; 7% overall), whereas most cancers identified were localized. Only 14% of invasive procedures were carried out for benign disease.

The ongoing UK Lung Cancer Screening Trial[28] recognizes 4 nodule categories adding nodule shape and relation to pleura, size, and volume.

The utility of PET-CT in nodule management was investigated by the author's group[29,30] and the Danish group.[31] The author's group found that PET-CT sensitivity at baseline was 88% overall and 100% for solid nodules greater than 1 cm. For incident nodules, however, overall sensitivity fell sharply to less than 60%.[30] The Danish group[31] had similar experience with PET-CT but found that a combination of VDT and PET-CT produced good sensitivity and specificity.

ONCOLOGIC OUTCOMES

Randomized trials conducted in North America and Europe have attempted to address the contentious issue of whether lung cancer screening can reduce mortality.[6,32–34] Although the US NLST[6] was designed with sufficient power to demonstrate a benefit of screening, sample sizes in most European trials were low and statistical power was insufficient to demonstrate any mortality benefit. The European NELSON study was an exception and is expected to release results after 2015.

Three European screening trials—the Detection and Screening of Early Lung Cancer by Novel Imaging Technology and Molecular Essays (DANTE) study,[32] the DLCST,[34] and the Multicentric Italian Lung Detection (MILD) study[33]—have published mortality findings; none found a mortality reduction in the screened arm.

In DANTE, all participants received baseline chest radiograph and were then randomized to either LDCT screening or usual care. Analysis after 3 years revealed no significant difference in all-cause or lung cancer–specific mortality between the screened and control arms (**Fig. 3**) (2.0% vs 2.1% and 1.6% vs 1.7%, respectively).[32] Any mortality reduction, however, is only likely to become evident beyond 3 years. It is also noteworthy that the proportion of stage I cancers in the screened arm was lower in DANTE than in other studies, and rate of interval cancers was higher, possibly because an outmoded single-slice CT was used, and criteria for surgical resection were more restrictive than in other studies. The more advanced age of the DANTE study population and longer observation period could also have played a role. Finally, because only men were recruited, and all received baseline chest radiograph, DANTE findings may not be generalizable.

The DLCST[34] found no reduction in lung cancer or all-cause mortality after 5 screening rounds. The investigators suggested this was due to small sample size and short follow-up. After a median follow-up of 4.8 years, relative risks (RRs) were 1.37 (95% CI, 0.63–2.97) for lung cancer mortality and 1.46 (95% CI, 0.99–2.15) for all-cause mortality in the screened group.

The MILD study[33] is a single-center trial comparing annual or biennial LDCT with no lung cancer screening. All-cause mortality did not differ significantly between the combined screening groups and control group (RR 1.40; 95% CI, 0.82–2.38). When the annual LDCT group was compared with the control group, however, RR for all-cause mortality was 1.80.

Nonrandomized (single-arm) studies have also analyzed oncological outcomes.[35] The author's group in Milan presented results of 11 years of active annual screening in 2010[35] and found that the cancer rate was stable over time—evidence against hypothesized overdiagnosis and depletion of cancer cases after the first 2 to 3 years; even the proportion of early stage disease remained stable over time. Lung cancer mortality in this cohort was less than in an age- and gender-matched population of US smokers, suggesting that mortality can be lowered by screening. The author's group in estimated a 50% mortality reduction after 7 years of annual screening.[35] **Fig. 4** summarizes the results of mortality analyses from the randomized trials available so far.[10]

Table 1
Results of selected modern lung cancer screening trials

Study	Started	N[a]	Age	Baseline Low-Dose CT Screen Percentage Abnormal[a]	LC	Percentage	N[a] of Rounds	Overall (with Incidence Screens) Total LC	Percentage	Stage I	Percentage
Shinshu Uni	1996	5483	40–74	5	23	0.42	3	63	1.1	51	81
Hitachi	1998	7965	50–69	26	36	0.44	2	40	0.05	31	78
Milan	2000	1035	50–84	21	11	1.06	2	22	2.1	16	73
Pamplona	2000	911	>40	48	12	1.32	2	14	1.5	13	93
Mayo Clinic	1998	1520	50–85	51	27	1.78	5	66	4.5	36	55
I-ELCAP	1994	31,567	40–85	13	405	41.28	2	484	1.5	412	485
Milan Uni	2004	5189	>50	10	55	1.04	2	92	1.8	61	66
PLuSS	2002	3642	50–79	40	53	1.45	2	80	2.2	40	50
Toronto	2003	3352	50–83	18	56	1.67	2	65	1.9	42	65

Total LC, all cases detected throughout the study period, including interval cases.
Abbreviation: LC, patients diagnosed with lung cancer.
[a] Patients with any abnormality in their baseline CT scan.
Adapted from Nair A, Hansell DM. European and North American lung cancer screening experience and implications for pulmonary nodule management. Eur Radiol 2011;21(12):2447.

Table 2
Summary data for the COSMOS screening study over 5 years

Screening Round	Total Participants N (%)	Recalled for CT or PET N (%)	Recalled for PET N (%)	First Primary Lung Cancer N (%)	Localized Cancer (N0M0) N (%)	Mean Size mm (SD)	PET-Positive N (%)	Nonsolid Nodule N (%)
Baseline	5203 (100)	525 (10.1)	160 (3.1)	55 (1.06)	43 (78.2)	20.6 (13.6)	48 (87.3)	4 (7.3)
2nd	4822 (93)	189 (3.9)	68 (1.4)	38 (0.79)	26 (68.4)	13.6 (7.2)	26 (68.4)	5 (13.2)
3rd	4583 (88)	232 (5.1)	74 (1.6)	39 (0.85)	34 (87.2)	12.4 (7.5)	11 (28.2)	13 (33.3)
4th	4385 (84)	289 (6.6)	62 (1.4)	31 (0.71)	23 (74.2)	18.6 (18.6)	21 (67.7)	6 (19.4)
5th	4123 (79)	241 (5.8)	66 (1.6)	12 (0.29)	10 (83.3)	11.0 (4.5)	5 (41.7)	2 (16.7)
Whole period	(23,116 person-years of observation)	1476 (6.4)	430 (1.9)	175 (0.76)	136 (77.7)	16.2 (12.5)	111 (63.4)	30 (17.1)

From Veronesi G, Maisonneuve P, Spaggiari L, et al. Diagnostic performance of low-dose computed tomography screening for lung cancer over 5 years. J Thorac Oncol 2014;9(7):936; with permission.

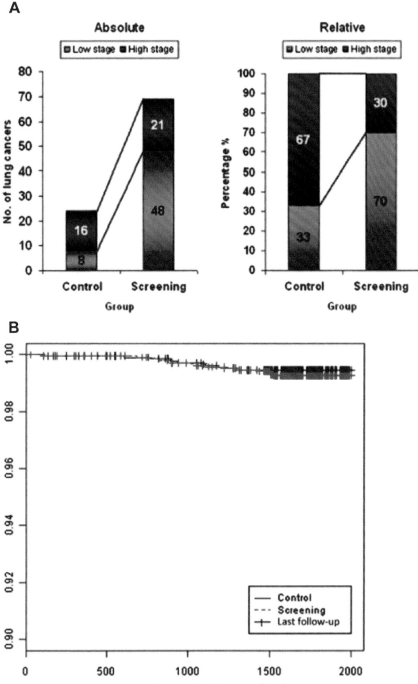

Fig. 3. (A) Absolute number of lung cancers detected in the control and screening arms in DANTE study and relative distribution according to stage at diagnosis. (B) Survival curve of the entire population according to the arm of randomization. (*Data from* Infante M, Cavuto S, Lutman FR, et al. A randomized study of lung cancer screening with spiral computed tomography: 3-year results from the DANTE trial. Am J Respir Crit Care Med 2009;180(5):445–53.)

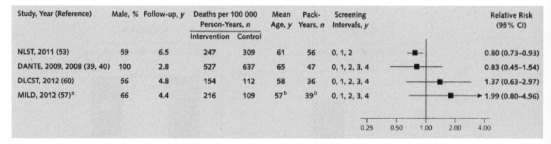

Study, Year (Reference)	Male, %	Follow-up, y	Deaths per 100 000 Person-Years, n		Mean Age, y	Pack-Years, n	Screening Intervals, y	Relative Risk (95% CI)
			Intervention	Control				
NLST, 2011 (53)	59	6.5	247	309	61	56	0, 1, 2	0.80 (0.73–0.93)
DANTE, 2009, 2008 (39, 40)	100	2.8	527	637	65	47	0, 1, 2, 3, 4	0.83 (0.45–1.54)
DLCST, 2012 (60)	56	4.8	154	112	58	36	0, 1, 2, 3, 4	1.37 (0.63–2.97)
MILD, 2012 (57)[a]	66	4.4	216	109	57[b]	39[b]	0, 1, 2, 3, 4	1.99 (0.80–4.96)

Fig. 4. Trial results for lung cancer mortality. [a] Annual screening group compared only with control group; biennial screening group not shown. [b] Median. (*From* Humphrey LL, Deffebach M, Pappas M, et al. Screening for lung cancer with low-dose computed tomography: a systematic review to update the US Preventive services task force recommendation. Ann Intern Med 2013;159(6):411–20; with permission.)

TREATMENT OF SCREENING-DETECTED LUNG CANCERS

European studies published in 2014[23] and 2012[36] indicate that the mean size of screening-detected lung cancers is approximately 16 mm, approximately 30% of which have long VDTs (more than 400 days), suggesting relatively nonaggressive disease. These findings suggest a need to investigate treatments that are less aggressive than the standard approach, which is lung lobectomy plus mediastinal and hilar lymphadenectomy and may be overtreatment for small peripheral cancers often shown to be without mediastinal or hilar lymph node involvement. Segmental resections[37] and stereotactic ablative radiotherapy[38,39] are under evaluation in prospective randomized studies. The surgery itself has also become less invasive as video-assisted thoracic surgery (VATS)[40] and robotic surgery[41] are being used, in some centers, instead of thoracotomy.

The author's group's experience is that approximately 10% of patients with screening-detected lung cancer develop a new primary lung cancer in the 5 years after treatment.[23] Such patients do not easily tolerate second conventional surgery and would perhaps be better served by sublobar resection VATS or robotic surgery for both surgeries or at least the second. It is encouraging that the Danish group[40] reported that proportionately more patients with screening-detected cancer underwent VATS than patients whose lung cancer was detected outside a screening program.

Regarding lymph node dissection, there is no consensus as to whether this should be performed for subcentimeter lung cancers. The author's group retrospectively assessed 219 patients with pathologic T1 non–small cell lung cancer (NSCLC), staged by high-resolution CT and PET as stage I, who underwent anatomic resection and radical lymphadenectomy[42,43] and found that cases of tumor less than 1 cm or of glucose uptake (standardized uptake value) less than 2 had very low probability of nodal involvement, suggesting that lymphadenectomy could be avoided in such cases. By contrast, cancers greater than 1 cm in diameter had 20% rate of occult lymph node involvement even though N0 at preoperative staging.

Stereotactic radiation therapy is an established modality for the local treatment of primary and secondary thoracic lesions.[44] For primary lung cancer, the technique is now considered the first alternative to surgery in patients who are medically inoperable due to insufficient cardiac or pulmonary reserve. Stereotactic radiation is noninvasive, has a low toxicity profile, and is effective.[41–44] Prospective investigations are required, however, to assess its role in the treatment of stage Ia screening-detected cancers in fit patients.

MOLECULAR MARKERS FOR THE EARLY DETECTION OF LUNG CANCER

A blood test able to reliably detect early lung cancer would be an ideal tool for population-based lung cancer screening. In recent years there have been many attempts to identify serum/plasma biomarkers for lung cancer. Some studies have investigated ELISA to detect circulating tumor-associated antigens, such as p53, NY-ESO-1, CAGE, GBU 4–5, annexins, and SOX2, with moderately encouraging results.[45] Others have detected circulating cancer cells in the blood of patients with metastatic cancers[46] suggesting the utility of investigations to detect circulating cancer cells at earlier disease stages.

In 2011, a distinct subset of circulating micro-RNAs (miRNAs) was identified in symptomatic lung cancer cases.[47,48] More promisingly, 2 Italian centers were able to detect miRNAs indicative of LDCT-detected asymptomatic lung cancers.[11,49] Circulating miRNAs are an attractive alternative to LDCT for the early diagnosis of lung cancer, because they are easily quantified by real-time

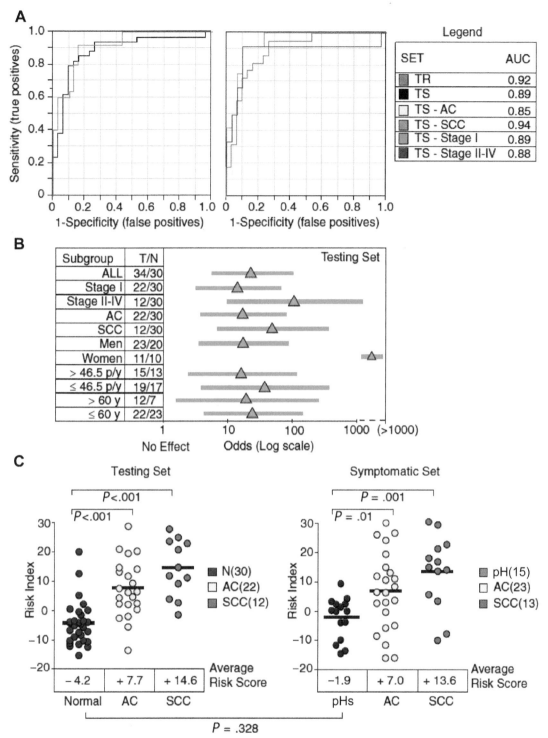

Fig. 5. The 34-miRNA diagnostic model. (*A*) Receiver operating characteristic curves of the 34-miRNA diagnostic model. Color codes are as per the legend. AC, adenocarcinoma; SCC, squamous cell carcinoma; TR, training set; TS, testing set; TS - AC, testing set considering only ACs; TS - SCC, testing set considering only SCCs; TS - Stage I, testing set considering only stage I tumors; TS - Stage II-IV, testing set considering all other tumor stages. (*B*) Forest plot showing the 34-miRNA model prediction strength in the testing set (all, 30 normal and 34 tumors) stratified by available clinical-pathologic parameters. Triangles represent the odds ratios; lines represent the relative 95% CIs (nominal logistic regression). Age (y) and packs/year (p/y) cutoffs were defined by the relative averages in the 64 patients. *P* values were less than 0.01 in all analyses (2-tailed Fisher exact test). (*C*) Risk of cancer based on the 34-miRNA risk model in NSCLC patients (separately for ACs and SCCs) from the testing set (*left panel*) and symptomatic cases (*right panel*). Average risk scores and *P* value (analysis of variance) are also shown. (*Data from* Bianchi F, Hu J, Pelosi G, et al. Lung cancers detected by screening with spiral computed tomography have a malignant phenotype when analyzed by cDNA microarray. Clin Cancer Res 2004;10(18 Pt 1):6023–8.)

polymerase chain reaction (PCR) and are fairly stable.[49,50] Real-time PCR was used to identify miRNA expression profiles from the serum of COSMOS study participants.[11] Of the 147 miRNAs detected, 34 differed in expression between persons with asymptomatic LDCT-detected lung adenocarcinoma and those without lung cancer (**Fig. 5**). A multivariate risk predictor algorithm was developed based on a weighted linear combination of expression levels of the 34 miRNAs. When the predictor was tested on an independent cohort of patients with asymptomatic LDCT-detected lung cancer, it had an overall accuracy of 80% (sensitivity 71%, specificity 90%; area under the curve [AUC] 0.89). The algorithm was able to distinguish between LDCT-detected benign nodules and frankly malignant disease. This latter finding is particularly interesting in view of the high numbers of indeterminate lung nodules detected by screening.

RISK MODELS

It is important to identify the best target population for screening and the optimal screening interval, to spare low-risk persons useless irradiation and contain screening costs. With the aim of assessing these issues, a UK group developed the Liverpool Lung Project (LLP) prediction model to estimate the probability that an individual, with a specified combination of risk factors, would develop lung cancer within a 5-year period.[51] They used a

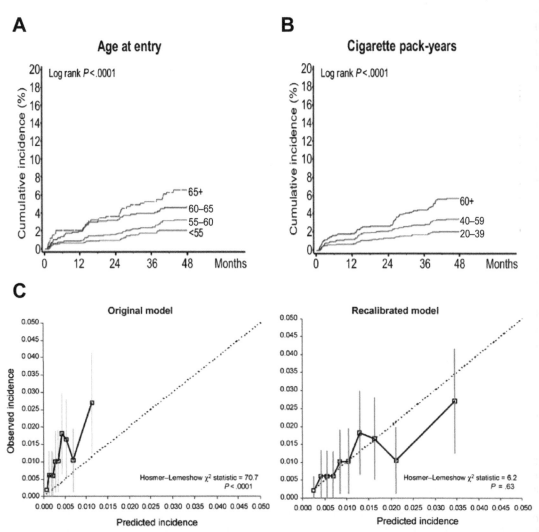

Fig. 6. Correlation between the cumulative incidence of lung cancer in the COSMOS study and the 2 most important risk factors, (A) age and (B) smoking (pack-years). (C) The Bach model was recalibrated in the COSMOS risk model, to adapt the risk to a screening population. (From Maisonneuve P, Bagnardi V, Bellomi M, et al. Lung Cancer Risk Prediction to Select Smokers for Screening CT–a Model Based on the Italian COSMOS Trial. Cancer Prev Res (Phila) 2011;4(11):1778–89; with permission.)

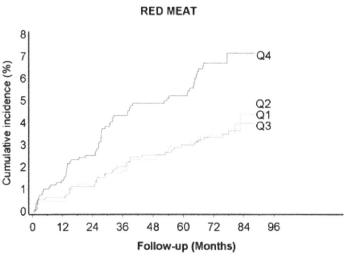

Fig. 7. Cumulative incidence of lung cancers detected through repeated annual screening CT scans according to daily quartile food density of red meat and olive oil and according to average daily tea and wine consumption. (*Adapted from* Gnagnarella P, Maisonneuve P, Bellomi M, et al. Red meat, Mediterranean diet and lung cancer risk among heavy smokers in the COSMOS screening study. Ann Oncol 2013;24(10):2606–11.)

training set of 579 lung cancers patients and 1157 controls. Choosing the 2.5% probability of developing lung cancer as cutoff to trigger increased surveillance gave a sensitivity of 0.62 and specificity of 0.70, whereas a 6.0% cutoff gave a sensitivity of 0.34 and specificity of 0.90. The classification power for the model was assessed by a 10-fold cross-validation procedure, and analysis of receiver operating characteristics (AUC calculations). The analysis showed gave an AUC of 0.70 indicating good discrimination. The model must be validated, however, on a new set of patients and controls.

The COSMOS study was the first to develop a lung cancer risk model for specific use in the screening context.[52] The model was able to select subjects for initial screening and define the optimal screening interval for individuals being screened, based on personal characteristics. To choose subjects for screening, the model includes the 2 most important risk factors age and smoking (pack-years) (**Fig. 6**). After evaluating several other variables in univariate and multivariate analyses, the variables of the Bach model[53] were found the most effective for selecting who should be screened and were incorporated into a new recalibrated Bach model.

To assess optimal screening interval, nodule characteristics at baseline were incorporated into the model to assess the risk of developing cancer after baseline screening. The model classifies the screened population into 5 risk groups. The very low risk group was considered to require screening every 2 to 3 years, whereas the high-risk group was considered to require fairly intensive surveillance. Application of the model may reduce the number of LDCT scans required to detect 1 cancer.

The results of a recent epidemiologic analysis of nutrition in heavy smokers who participated in an Italian LDCT screening program suggested that high adherence to a Mediterranean diet in the year preceding enrollment was associated with lower detection of lung cancers in asymptomatic heavy smokers.[54] The validated self-administered food frequency questionnaire (FFQ) developed for the Italian component of the European Prospective Investigation into Cancer and Nutrition study was distributed to the 5203 participants of the COSMOS study.[55] Completed FFQs were returned by 4336 (84%). Analysis indicated that a diet rich in fruits and vegetables, with olive oil as main source of fat, moderate consumption of wine, and low consumption of red meat, was responsible for the risk reduction (**Fig. 7**). Physicians and health care providers should include nutrition in educational campaigns to promote a healthy lifestyle.

SUMMARY

Lung cancer is a rapidly fatal disease that claims the lives of more people annually than the next 4 most lethal cancers combined (in order, colon, breast, pancreatic, and prostate cancers). After the publication of the NLST results in November 2011, confidence that lung cancer screening could be effective soared, and approximately 40 scientific societies subsequently endorsed LDCT screening.

In the United States, the implementation of LDCT screening is progressing rapidly. In December 2013, the US Preventive Services Task Force endorsed LDCT and US health insurance companies have started to cover it. In July 2014, the US Centers for Medicare and Medicaid Services released a new S code for LDCT lung cancer screening and will probably vote in favor of LDCT coverage even though, in April 2014, the Medicare Evidence Development and Coverage Advisory Committee concluded that there was not enough evidence to justify annual LDCT screening for the detection of early lung cancer.

In Europe, large-scale implementation of LDCT screening faces many obstacles, and there is widespread doubt as to its benefit, mainly because the several underpowered randomized trials conducted in Europe failed to demonstrate a mortality reduction in the screened arm compared with the control arm. Furthermore, uncertainties as to how screening should be implemented have been voiced by several investigators, with questions, such as optimal screening interval, cutoff size for defining a positive nodule, and work-up algorithm, still to be resolved.

Despite these uncertainties, several European centers have pushed ahead with screening protocols developed and refined in house. Encouraging results have also been obtained on biomarkers in serum to diagnose very early cancer: these have potential for the definition of screened populations and for incorporation into risk models.

Important advances have also been made in nodule work-up algorithms and surgical treatments. Randomized trials to compare limited resection versus lobectomy are ongoing in Europe to determine whether limited resection is appropriate for very early screening-detected cancers.

To ensure the implementation of large-scale lung cancer screening in Europe, it will be important to create a coalition of European physicians, scientists, and health care providers to keep the issue before the public eye and combine it with the insistent message that stopping smoking is an effective means of preventing lung cancer—both independent of and in association with screening.

REFERENCES

1. Jemal A, Bray F, Center MM, et al. Global cancer statistics. CA Cancer J Clin 2011;61(2):69–90.
2. NCI: SEER Cancer Statistics Review, 1996-2002.
3. Diederich S, Thomas M, Semik M, et al. Screening for early lung cancer with low-dose spiral computed tomography: results of annual follow-up examinations in asymptomatic smokers. Eur Radiol 2004;14(4):691.
4. Henschke CI, McCauley DI, Yankelevitz DF, et al. Early Lung Cancer Action Project: overall design and findings from baseline screening. Lancet 1999;354(9173):99.
5. Sone S, Li F, Yang ZG, et al. Characteristics of small lung cancers invisible on conventional chest radiography and detected by population based screening using spiral CT. Br J Radiol 2000;73(866):137.
6. Aberle DR, Adams AM, Berg CD, et al. Reduced lung-cancer mortality with low-dose computed tomographic screening. N Engl J Med 2011; 365(5):395–409.
7. McMahon PM, Kong CY, Johnson BE, et al. Estimating long-term effectiveness of lung cancer screening in the Mayo CT Screening Study. Radiology 2008;248:278–87.
8. Chien CR, His TH. Mean sojourn time and effectiveness of mortality reduction for lung cancer screening with computed tomography. Int J Cancer 2008;122: 2594–9.
9. American Society of Clinical Oncology. The Role of CT Screening for Lung Cancer in Clinical Practice. The Evidence Based Practice Guideline of the American College of Chest Physicians and the American Society for Clinical Oncology. Available at: www.asco.org/quality-guidelines/role-ct-screening-lung-cancer-clinical-practice-evidencebased-practice-guideline. Accessed January 23, 2014. May 20, 2012.
10. Humphrey LL, Deffebach M, Pappas M, et al. Screening for lung cancer with low-dose computed tomography: a systematic review to update the U.S. Preventive Services Task Force Recommendation. Ann Intern Med 2013;159:411–20.
11. Boeri M, Verri C, Conte D, et al. MicroRNA signatures in tissues and plasma predict development and prognosis of computed tomography detected lung cancer. Proc Natl Acad Sci U S A 2011;108:3713–8.
12. Bianchi F, Hu J, Pelosi G, et al. Lung cancers detected by screening with spiral computed tomography have a malignant phenotype when analyzed by cDNA microarray. Clin Cancer Res 2004;10(18 Pt 1):6023–8.
13. Field JK, Oudkerk M, Pedersen JH, et al. Prospects for population screening and diagnosis of lung cancer. Lancet 2013;382(9893):732–41.
14. Centers for Disease Control and Prevention. Lung cancer: risk factors. Available at: http://www.cdc.gov/cancer/lung/basic_info/risk_factors.htm. Accessed July 1, 2013.
15. US Department of Health and Human Services, Centers for Disease Control and Prevention and Health Promotion, Office on Smoking and Health. The Health Consequences of Smoking—50 Years of Progress: A Report of the Surgeon General. Washington, DC: USDHSS; 2014. p. 4–20.

16. Ashraf H, Tønnesen P, Holst Pedersen J, et al. Effect of CT screening on smoking habits at 1-year follow-up in the Danish Lung Cancer Screening Trial (DLCST). Thorax 2009;64:388–92.

17. van der Aalst CM, van den Bergh KA, Willemsen MC, et al. Lung cancer screening and smoking abstinence: 2 year follow-up data from the Dutch-Belgian randomised controlled lung cancer screening trial. Thorax 2010;65(7):600–5.

18. van der Aalst CM, de Koning HJ, van den Bergh KA, et al. The effectiveness of a computer-tailored smoking cessation intervention for participants in lung cancer screening: a randomised controlled trial. Lung Cancer 2012;76(2):204–10.

19. Keith RL, Miller YE. Lung cancer chemoprevention: current status and future prospects. Nat Rev Clin Oncol 2013;10:334–43.

20. Veronesi G, Szabo E, Decensi A, et al. Randomized phase II trial of inhaled budesonide versus placebo in high-risk individuals with CT screen-detected lung nodules. Cancer Prev Res (Phila) 2011;4:34–42.

21. Rothwell PM, Fowkes FG, Belch JF, et al. Effect of daily aspirin on long-term risk of death due to cancer: analysis of individual patient data from randomised trials. Lancet 2011;377(9759): 31–41.

22. Cuzick J, Thorat MA, Bosetti C, et al. Estimates of benefits and harms of prophylactic use of aspirin in the general population. Ann Oncol 2014.

23. Veronesi G, Maisonneuve P, Spaggiari L, et al. Diagnostic performance of low-dose computed tomography screening for lung cancer over five years. J Thorac Oncol 2014;9(7):935–9.

24. International Early Lung Cancer Action Program Investigators. Survival of patients with stage I lung cancer detected on CT screening. N Engl J Med 2006;355(17):1763–71.

25. Available at: http://seer.cancer.gov/statfacts/html/lungb.html. Accessed July 1, 2013.

26. van Klaveren RJ, Oudkerk M, Prokop M, et al. Management of lung nodules detected by volume CT scanning. N Engl J Med 2009;361(23):2221–9.

27. Nair A, Hansell DM. European and North American lung cancer screening experience and implications for pulmonary nodule management. Eur Radiol 2011;21(12):2445–54.

28. Baldwin DR, Duffy SW, Wald NJ, et al. UK Lung Screen (UKLS) nodule management protocol: modelling of a single screen randomised controlled trial of low-dose CT screening for lung cancer. Thorax 2011;66(4):308–13.

29. Veronesi G, Bellomi M, Veronesi U, et al. Role of positron emission tomography scanning in the management of lung nodules detected at baseline computed tomography screening. Ann Thorac Surg 2007;84:959–65.

30. Veronesi G, Travaini LL, Maisonneuve P, et al. Positron emission tomography in the diagnostic work-up of screening-detected lung nodules. Eur Respir J 2014. [Epub ahead of print].

31. Ashraf H, Dirksen A, Loft A, et al. Combined use of positron emission tomography and volume doubling time in lung cancer screening with low-dose CT scanning. Thorax 2011;66:315–9.

32. Infante M, Cavuto S, Lutman FR, et al. A randomized study of lung cancer screening with spiral computed tomography: three-year results from the DANTE trial. Am J Respir Crit Care Med 2009; 180(5):445–53.

33. Pastorino U, Rossi M, Rosato V, et al. Annual or biennial CT screening versus observation in heavy smokers: 5-year results of the MILD trial. Eur J Cancer Prev 2012;21(3):308–15.

34. Saghir Z, Dirksen A, Ashraf H, et al. CT screening for lung cancer brings forward early disease. The randomised Danish Lung Cancer Screening Trial: status after five annual screening rounds with low-dose. Thorax 2012;67(4):296–301.

35. Veronesi G, Maisonneuve P, Spaggiari L, et al. Long-term outcomes of a pilot CT screening for lung cancer. Ecancermedicalscience 2010;4:186.

36. Veronesi G, Maisonneuve P, Bellomi M, et al. Estimating overdiagnosis in low-dose computed tomography screening for lung cancer a cohort study. Ann Intern Med 2012;157(11):776–84.

37. Nakamura K, Saji H, Nakajima R, et al. Phase III randomised trial of lobectomy versus limited resection for small size peripheral NSCLC (JCOG0802/WJOG4607L). Jpn J Clin Oncol 2010;40:271–4.

38. Guckenberger M, Allgäuer M, Appold S, et al. Safety and efficacy of stereotactic body radiotherapy for stage 1 non-small-cell lung cancer in routine clinical practice: a patterns-of-care and outcome analysis. J Thorac Oncol 2013;8(8):1050–8.

39. Robinson CG, DeWees TA, El Naqa IM, et al. Patterns of failure after stereotactic body radiation therapy or lobar resection for clinical stage I non-small-cell lung cancer. J Thorac Oncol 2013; 8:192–201.

40. Petersen RH, Hansen HJ, Dirksen A, et al. Lung cancer screening and video-assisted thoracic surgery. J Thorac Oncol 2012;7(6):1026–31.

41. Veronesi G, Galetta D, Maisonneuve P, et al. Four-arm robotic lobectomy for the treatment of early-stage lung cancer. J Thorac Cardiovasc Surg 2010;140(1):19–25.

42. Veronesi G, Maisonneuve P, Pelosi G, et al. Screening-detected lung cancers: is systematic nodal dissection always essential? J Thorac Oncol 2011;6(3):525–30.

43. Casiraghi M, Travaini LL, Maisonneuve P, et al. Lymph node involvement in T1 non-small-cell lung cancer: could glucose uptake and maximal

diameter be predictive criteria? Eur J Cardiothorac Surg 2011;39(4):e38–43.

44. Senan S, Paul MA, Lagerwaard FJ. Treatment of early-stage lung cancer detected by screening: surgery or stereotactic ablative radiotherapy? Lancet Oncol 2013;14(7):e270–4.

45. Maheswaran S, Sequist LV, Nagrath S, et al. Detection of mutations in EGFR in circulating lung-cancer cells. N Engl J Med 2008;359(4):366–77.

46. Shen J, Todd NW, Zhang H, et al. Plasma microRNAs as potential biomarkers for non-small-cell lung cancer. Lab Invest 2011;91:579–87.

47. Zheng D, Haddadin S, Wang Y, et al. Plasma microRNAs as novel biomarkers for early detection of lung cancer. Int J Clin Exp Pathol 2011;4:575–86.

48. Bianchi F, Nicassio F, Marzi M, et al. A serum circulating miRNA diagnostic test to identify asymptomatic high-risk individuals with early stage lung cancer. EMBO Mol Med 2011;3:495–503.

49. Chen X, Ba Y, Ma L. Characterization of microRNAs in serum: a novel class of biomarkers for diagnosis of cancer and other diseases. Cell Res 2008; 18(10):997–1006.

50. Valadi H, Ekström K, Bossios A, et al. Exosome-mediated transfer of mRNAs and microRNAs is a novel mechanism of genetic exchange between cells. Nat Cell Biol 2007;9(6):654–9.

51. Cassidy A, Myles JP, van Tongeren M, et al. The LLP risk model: an individual risk prediction model for lung cancer. Br J Cancer 2008;98:270–6.

52. Maisonneuve P, Bagnardi V, Bellomi M, et al. Lung Cancer Risk Prediction to Select Smokers for Screening CT–a Model Based on the Italian COSMOS Trial. Cancer Prev Res (Phila) 2011; 4(11):1778–89.

53. Bach PB, Kattan MW, Thornquist MD, et al. Variations in lung cancer risk among smokers. J Natl Cancer Inst 2003;95:470–8.

54. Gnagnarella P, Maisonneuve P, Bellomi M, et al. Red meat, Mediterranean diet and lung cancer risk among heavy smokers in the COSMOS screening study. Ann Oncol 2013;24(10):2606–11.

55. Slimani N, Deharveng G, Charrondiere RU, et al. Structure of the standardized computerized 24-h diet recall interview used as reference method in the 22 centers participating in the EPIC project. European Prospective Investigation into Cancer and Nutrition. Comput Methods Programs Biomed 1999;58:251–66.

Surgeons and Lung Cancer Screening
Rules of Engagement

Sean C. Grondin, MD, MPH, FRCSC[a],*, Janet P. Edwards, MD, MPH, FRCSC[a],
Gaetano Rocco, MD, FRCS (Ed), FETCS[b]

KEYWORDS

- Lung • Cancer • Low-dose • CT • Screening • Surgeon • Program • Thoracic

KEY POINTS

- To understand the challenges of screening for lung cancer, surgeons should be familiar with the fundamental epidemiologic concepts pertaining to screening and have an understanding of the evidence regarding the various modalities used in screening for lung cancer.
- A recent study has confirmed that screening for lung cancer with low-dose computed tomography (CT) decreases mortality in high-risk individuals.
- High-quality programs should be safe and cost-effective as well as accessible to all high-risk patients and involve the participation of a multidisciplinary team.
- Surgeons need to be actively engaged in the implementation of CT screening programs as well as have input on the design of diagnostic and therapeutic decision-making algorithms.
- Thoracic surgeons should actively participate in the CT screening program in order to optimize the management of screen-detected lung nodules.

INTRODUCTION

Lung cancer is the most common cancer and the largest contributor to cancer mortality worldwide, with more than 1.8 million incident cases and 1.6 million attributable deaths in 2012.[1] In the United States alone, there will be a projected 224,210 new cases and 159,260 lung cancer deaths in 2014 representing 27% of all cancer deaths in the United States.[2] The mortality rate of lung cancer is extremely high, with a case fatality rate of 87%.[1] In patients diagnosed with lung cancer, the overall 5-year survival is reported in the realm of 15%.[3]

The dismal survival seen with lung cancer is in part caused by the large proportion of patients who present with locally advanced or metastatic disease. The 15% of patients with lung cancer who present with disease localized to the primary site experience 54% survival at 5 years. Unfortunately, advanced disease at the time of diagnosis is much more common, with 22% of patients presenting with regional lymph node involvement and 57% presenting with distant metastases. The 5-year survival in these groups is substantially worse at 26% and 4%, respectively.[4] Given this, the potential for screening to improve early

The authors have nothing to disclose.
[a] Department of Surgery, Foothills Medical Centre, University of Calgary, 1403 29th Street Northwest, Room G 33 D, Calgary, Alberta T2N 2T9, Canada; [b] Division of Thoracic Surgery, Department of Thoracic Surgery and Oncology, Istituto Nazionale Tumori, Fondazione Pascale, IRCCS, Naples, Napoli, Italy
* Corresponding author.
E-mail address: sean.grondin@albertahealthservices.ca

Thorac Surg Clin 25 (2015) 175–184
http://dx.doi.org/10.1016/j.thorsurg.2014.11.004

detection and reduce mortality has been the subject of much investigation.

EPIDEMIOLOGY OF SCREENING

Screening has been defined as

> *The presumptive identification of unrecognized disease or defect by the application of tests, examinations, or other procedures which can be applied rapidly to sort out apparently well persons who probably have a disease from those who probably do not. A screening test is not intended to be diagnostic. Persons with positive or suspicious findings must be referred to their physicians for diagnosis and necessary treatment.[5]*

The central assumption underlying the presumed utility of any screening program is that prognosis is improved by early detection and treatment of a given disease at an asymptomatic stage.[6]

The development and implementation of screening programs is a complex endeavor. Although the aim is to improve health, such interventions may also have the potential to harm the health of individuals or negatively impact the economic health of a nation. Therefore, it is important to take a principled approach to the implementation and evaluation of screening programs. The seminal publication by Wilson and Jungner[7] enumerated the principles of early disease detection or screening (**Box 1**). These principles provide a structured approach to follow when designing a screening program. If these conditions are not met, the benefits of implementing a proposed screening program should be questioned.

It is essential that screening programs be evaluated in a similarly principled manner. Factors contributing to the overall evaluation of screening programs include validity, reliability, feasibility, and effectiveness.[6] Each of these criteria is summarized briefly next.

1. *Validity*: The better the test, the higher its ability to accurately classify as positive those with a disease (sensitivity) and to classify as negative those without a disease (specificity). There is often a trade-off between these two measures of validity, erring toward increased sensitivity when the repercussions of missing a case of disease are high (as with a highly fatal disease) and increased specificity if the further steps required to establish a diagnosis are invasive or potentially harmful.
2. *Reliability*: Reliable tests provide consistent, repeatable results when performed in similar patients under comparable conditions. Reliability is influenced by the dependence of the test result on interpretation by the operator, the variability of the feature being measured in a given patient, as well as the consistency of the tool being used for measurement.
3. *Feasibility*: This feature is complex and is often difficult to quantify with one or a small number of measures. It involves acceptability of the testing program to the public, the cost

---

Box 1
The principles of early disease detection or screening

1. The condition sought should be an important health problem.
2. There should be an accepted treatment of patients with recognized disease.
3. Facilities for diagnosis and treatment should be available.
4. There should be a recognizable latent stage, referred to elsewhere as a detectable preclinical stage of disease.
5. There should be a suitable test or examination.
6. The test should be acceptable to the population.
7. The natural history of the condition, including development from latent to declared disease, should be adequately understood.
8. There should be an agreed policy on whom to treat as patients.
9. The cost of case finding (including diagnosis and treatment of patients diagnosed) should be economically balanced in relation to possible expenditure on medical care as a whole.
10. Case finding should be a continuing process and not a once-and-for-all project.

From Wilson JM, Jungner F. Principles and practice of screening for disease (Public Health Papers No. 34). Geneva (Switzerland): WHO; 1968. Available at: http://whqlibdoc.who.int/php/WHO_PHP_34.pdf. Accessed July 17, 2014.

and availability of the screening test, and the cost and availability of subsequent testing and treatment. One measure that contributes to an understanding of feasibility is yield, which can be calculated in terms of the predictive value of the test. The positive predictive value indicates the probability that an individual truly has the disease given a positive test result, whereas the negative predictive value indicates the probability that an individual with a negative test result does not have the disease.

4. *Effectiveness*: This feature refers to whether the screening program being evaluated accomplishes the ultimate goal of reducing morbidity and mortality from the disease. According to Hennekens and Buring,[7] "the most definitive measure of the efficacy of a screening program is a comparison of the cause-specific mortality rates among those whose disease was picked up by screening and those whose diagnosis was related to the development of symptoms." Baseline imbalances between these two groups often complicate such a comparison as volunteers for screening programs may be healthier and more compliant with investigation and treatment regimens. Conversely, they may be at higher risk of the disease and choose to participate because of family history, for example. Lead-time and length-time bias also confound the interpretation of data comparing screened and unscreened populations. Lead-time bias refers to the time between detection within a screening program and when the disease would have become apparent without screening. Although survival may seem longer in unscreened populations, this can be caused at least in part by lead-time bias. Length-time bias refers to the possibility that those cases detected through screening may be more indolent than cases detected on clinical grounds; this less aggressive course of disease may erroneously suggest a benefit to screening. Length-time bias could therefore be a factor in lung cancer screening as the doubling time of lung cancers varies from 42 to 1486 days.[8]

LUNG CANCER SCREENING MODALITIES

Since the 1970s, various modalities have been investigated as potential methods to improve early detection of lung cancer and potentially improve prognosis. The main modalities that have been explored include chest radiograph (CXR), sputum cytology, and low-dose chest computed tomography (CT). These modalities are described later along with a summary of the evidence for the efficacy of each method, focusing on randomized controlled trials.

Chest Radiograph

There has been one recent, very large study randomizing 154,901 men and women aged 55 to 74 years to annual CXR screening or usual care.[9] In the usual care group, no interventions were offered in addition to their standard medical care. Patients were not excluded based on smoking status, resulting in a similar but significant proportion of study participants in each group being never smokers (45.1% intervention, 44.2% usual care). There was no significant difference in lung cancer mortality for a median 11.9 years of follow-up in each group (relative risk [RR] 1.05, 95% confidence interval [CI] 0.87–1.12). Although the lung cancer incidence rates were higher when only smokers and former smokers were analyzed, there was still no significant difference between the intervention and usual care groups. Recent guidelines advise against the use of CXR for lung cancer screening because of a lack of proven benefit.[10]

Sputum Cytology

The ability of cytologic screening to reduce mortality from cervical cancer generated interest into the use of sputum cytology for lung cancer screening.[11] Two large randomized controlled trials have been conducted to explore the utility of screening for lung cancer using sputum cytology, specifically light microscopic cytomorphologic examination of exfoliated cells found in sputum samples.[12,13] Both of these studies, initiated in the 1970s, explored the incremental benefit of dual screening with CXR and sputum cytology compared with CXR alone in male current smokers of at least one pack per day, aged 45 years or greater with no previous history of lung cancer. The dual intervention was hypothesized to be superior to CXR alone as sputum would more likely detect central cancers, whereas CXR would more likely detect peripheral cancers.[14] The sputum analysis was carried out every 4 months in addition to yearly CXR for a follow-up period of 5 to 8 years. Neither study showed a statistically significant benefit to sputum analysis. In a pooled analysis of these two studies, totaling more than 20,000 patients, there was a nonsignificant trend toward reduced mortality from lung cancer in the intervention group (RR 0.88, 95% CI 0.74–1.03).[15] Recent guidelines advise against the use of sputum cytology for lung cancer screening because of a lack of proven benefit.[10]

Intensive Screening Using Both Chest Radiograph and Sputum Cytology

Several studies have evaluated the efficacy of intensive CXR screening versus less intensive radiographic screening. Some studies included sputum cytology in both arms, and some did not include it in either arm.[15–18] Although the inclusion criteria, follow-up, and frequency of investigations varied across studies, none showed a significant difference in mortality between the groups under study. Recent guidelines do not support intensive screening with CXR with or without sputum cytology.[10]

Low-Dose Chest Computed Tomography

There are several trials[19–26] evaluating CT as a method of screening for lung cancer, some of which are ongoing. The key features of these trials are detailed in **Table 1**. Importantly, the nature of

the control group varies between the American and European trials, with American trials using CXR in the control groups, whereas European studies using usual care.[27] **Table 2** highlights the results of those trials,[20,21,24,25] which have reported mortality outcomes from CT screening. Although the National Lung Screening Trial (NLST)[21] demonstrated a 20.0% relative reduction in mortality from lung cancer with low-dose CT screening (95% CI, 1.2–13.6, $P = .02$), none of the other trials[20,24,25] have reported a statistically significant difference in mortality between the CT screening and the controls arms. The size of the NLST far exceeds that of any other trial, powering it to detect differences in mortality that may not be seen with the smaller sample size of the other studies. Two factors may provide adequately powered data from the European studies: (1) the largest European trial has yet to report its mortality data,[22] and (2) the European studies could pool

Table 1
Design of randomized trials examining low-dose CT screening for lung cancer

Study	Year Started	Country	Number Enrolled	Age Range (y)	Smoking Requirement	Frequency of CTs	Control Group
LSS[19]	2000	United States	3318	55–74	Current or former min 30 pack y	Q1 y × 2	CXR
DANTE[20]	2001	Italy	2811	Men 60–74	Current or former min 20 pack y	Q1 y × 5	Observation
NLST[21]	2002	United States	53,454	55–74	Current or former min 30 pack y	Q1 y × 3	CXR
NELSON[22]	2003	Netherlands	15,822	50–74	Current and former smokers who smoked >15 cigarettes/d during >25 y or >10 cigarettes/d during >30 y	CT in y 1, 2, and 4	Observation
ITALUNG[23]	2004	Italy	3206	55–69	Current or former min 20 pack y	Q1 y × 4	Observation
DLCST[24]	2004	Denmark	4104	50–70	Current or former min 20 pack y	Q1 y × 5	Observation
MILD[25]	2005	Italy	4099	49+	Current or former min 20 pack y	2 Groups Q1 or Q2 y for 10 y	Observation
LUSI[26]	2007	Germany	4052	50–69	Heavy smoking	Q1 y × 5	Observation

Abbreviations: DANTE, detection and screening of early lung cancer trial; DLCST, Danish Lung Cancer Screening Trial; LSS, Lung Screening Study; MILD, multicentric italian lung detection; min, minimum; NELSON, dutch-belgian randomized lung cancer screening trial (Dutch acronym: NELSON study); NLST, National Lung Screening Trial.

Table 2
Randomized trials examining low-dose CT screening for lung cancer reporting mortality outcome

Study	Median Follow-up (y)	Cancers CT No. (%)	Cancers Control No. (%)	Lung Cancer Mortality CT No. (%)	Lung Cancer Mortality CT No. (%)	Lung Cancer–Specific Mortality Difference
DANTE[20]	2.8	60 (4.7)	34 (2.9)	20 (1.6)	20 (1.7)	$P = .84$
NLST[21]	6.5	1060 (4.0)	941 (3.5)	356 (1.3)	443 (1.7)	Risk reduction 20.0% (95% CI 6.8–26.7)
DLCST[24]	4.8	69 (3.4)	24 (1.2)	61 (3.0)	42 (2.1)	$P = .059$
MILD[25]	4.4	34 Annual CT (2.9) 25 Biennial CT (2.1)	20 (1.2)	12 Annual CT (1.0) 6 Biennial CT (0.5)	7 (4.1)	Hazard ratio 1.39 (95% CI 0.83–2.34)

Abbreviations: DANTE, detection and screening of early lung cancer trial; DLCST, Danish Lung Cancer Screening Trial; MILD, multicentric italian lung detection; NLST, National Lung Screening Trial.

their data into a meta-analysis once all of the studies have reported. A comprehensive discussion of the perspective from both American and Europe organizations as well as detailed results from key trials, such as NSLT, are discussed in other articles by Altorki, Wood, Allen, Blackmon, Jones Bach, and G Veronesi in this issue.

THE SURGEON'S ROLE IN OPTIMIZING COMPUTED TOMOGRAPHY SCREENING FOR LUNG CANCER

The optimal lung cancer CT screening program requires involvement of a multidisciplinary team that includes thoracic radiologists, pulmonologists, pathologists, medical and radiation oncologists, smoking cessation counselors, and thoracic surgeons. Thoracic surgeons should also be actively involved in both the design and implementation of a CT screening program in order to optimize the management of screen-detected lung nodules. Participating surgeons should be appropriately trained and credentialed in thoracic surgery and have expertise in lung cancer management. They should also provide expertise in the radiologic interpretation of lung nodules and recommendations for the appropriate diagnostic and therapeutic options available for surgical and nonsurgical patients. Furthermore, well-trained thoracic surgeons provide expertise in the preoperative evaluation of cardiopulmonary risk of patients and the analysis of surgical issues, such as the extent of resection, the need for mediastinal nodal dissection, and the management of synchronous lung nodules and ground-glass opacities. Finally, thoracic surgeons can determine whether the use of minimally invasive thoracic surgery techniques is the optimal approach for a given patient.[28]

As previously noted in this article, a large study has confirmed that screening for lung cancer with low-dose CT decreases mortality in high-risk individuals.[21] Although uncertainty exists about the generalizability, reproducibility, and potential bias of the trial results, decision makers and stakeholders, including patients and physicians, have become increasingly aware of the benefits of CT screening and are supportive of developing comprehensive screening programs.[8] In order to transition from CT screening trials to high-quality institutional or governmental CT screening programs, several important considerations need to be addressed. Thoracic surgeons need to be familiar with these challenges and be thoroughly involved in the planning and implementation of screening programs as well as being aware of the potential impact CT screening programs may have on workforce planning.[29]

High-Risk Population to Be Screened

Several surgical and nonsurgical organizations have endorsed screening with low-dose CT as an early detection technique that has the potential to significantly reduce lung cancer–related deaths.[30–35] However, in order to optimize resources and ensure a high-quality CT screening program for lung cancer, high-risk individuals who should be screened need to be accurately identified. Although the process of determining the appropriate individuals to be screened is in evolution, 2 high-risk groups who would benefit from screening have been identified.[31] Category 1 patients (aged 55–74 years, ≥30 pack year history of smoking, smoking cessation <15 years) have been selected based on high-level evidence, such as the NSLT trial. Category 2B patients (aged ≥50 years, ≥20 pack years of smoking, one additional risk factor other than smoking, such as exposure to radon, history of emphysema or pulmonary fibrosis, family history of lung cancer and other occupational exposure) are based on lower-level evidence.[31] In the NLST trial,[21] greater than 53,000 category 1 patients were screened with low-dose CT demonstrating a 20% reduction in lung cancer mortality. At this time, the appropriate age for screening remains controversial, with some groups recommending that screening guidelines should include patients older than 75 years.[30,36] Research is currently underway to refine high-risk populations for CT screening programs by studying comparative models and the variability of risk in patient populations using pooled data from studies with long-term follow-up.[37] The utility of CT screening for the routine follow-up of lung cancer surgery survivors is also currently being investigated.

Box 2
Fleischner Society's guidelines for the follow-up of incidentally discovered lung nodules in high-risk patients

Size of Nodule[a]	Follow-up Recommendations
≤4 mm	CT in 12 mo: if no growth, then no further follow-up
4–6 mm	CT in 6–12 mo, then 18 and 24 mo if no growth
6–8 mm	CT at 3–6 mo, then 9–12 mo, then 24 mo if no growth
>8 mm	CT at 3, 9, and 24 mo; PET and/or biopsy should be considered

[a] Size based on average of width and length.
Adapted from McMahon H, Austin JH, Gamsu G, et al. Guidelines for the management of small pulmonary nodules detected on CT scans: a systematic review from the Fleischner Society. Radiology 2005;237(2):398.

Duration and Frequency of Lung Cancer Screening

To date, the optimal duration of lung cancer screening has not been determined. In 2014, the National Comprehensive Cancer Network (NCCN) recommends that screening should continue for 3 years commencing up to and including 74 years of age. For instance, a patient starting screening at 55 years of age would be followed until 74 years of age, whereas an individual starting screening at 74 years of age would continue until 76 years of age.[31] No information is available on the benefits of screening high-risk patients annually for 25 to 30 years. Similarly, the impact on patients from the long-term exposure to radiation or potential investigation/treatment of nonmalignant nodules is not fully understood. These health risks are discussed in detail in the article by Dr Brian Meyers and colleagues in this issue.

The optimal frequency for screening high-risk patients requires further study in order to appropriately balance the benefits and health risks of CT screening as well as resource utilization and cost-effectiveness. Microsimulation modeling concluded that annual CT screening was most efficient when compared with biennial or triennial screening intervals.[38] In many centers, the recommendations for the evaluation of lung nodules adhere to the guidelines from the Fleischner Society, which are listed in **Box 2**.[39]

When establishing a CT screening program, concise guidelines for radiologists and clinicians are needed to define what constitutes a positive, negative, or indeterminate study. Successful implementation of a reporting system, such as the Lung Reporting and Data System (LU-RADS), will allow clear communication from the interpreting radiologists to the screening management team regarding the malignant potential of a nodules thereby ensuring appropriate testing or referrals.[40] Clear direction as to whom the patient is referred for follow-up for lung findings as well as nonlung findings, such as coronary artery calcification, is also needed.[41,42] The details of the follow-up process will depend on local practice guidelines and physician preference.

Minimizing of False-Positive Diagnoses

Careful selection of patients for surgery is essential to maximize the effectiveness of CT screening for lung cancer. In a review of several studies by Bach and colleagues,[43] approximately 20% of CT scans detect a suspicious nodule in each screening round, with 90% of these findings being benign. False-positive findings can result in unnecessary psychological distress, expense, and exposure to radiation. These results may also lead to unnecessary biopsies or surgeries that may in turn lead to morbidity and, in some cases, mortality. The surgical mortality reported in the NLST trial was 1%.[21]

Surgical morbidity is determined by the extent of the operative procedure and the rate of resection of benign disease. If surgery is necessary, video-assisted thoracoscopic surgery (VATS) wedge resection is the procedure of choice, where possible. Lobectomy for diagnosis should be performed as a procedure of last resort when other nonsurgical and minimally diagnostic modalities have failed. Currently, studies are underway to determine whether less extensive surgery, such as wedge resection or segmentectomy, may be adequate for resecting lung cancers of 2 cm or less.[44] With the judicious use of surgery, patients should realize the benefits of lung cancer treatment of tumors diagnosed at an earlier stage of disease.

When screening high-risk individuals with CT, the frequency of detecting a benign lung nodule varies depending on the characteristics of the screened population and the overall performance of the diagnostic algorithm used in the research protocol. In some reviews, the probability of detecting a benign pulmonary lesion on low-dose CT is 20 times higher than lung cancer detection rates.[27] A recent systematic review of major published studies concluded that surgical biopsies were indicated in more than 5% of nodules detected during CT screening, of which 0.5% to 4.5% were found to be cancer.[43] Furthermore, the investigators reported that on average surgical interventions resulted in a benign lesion in 25% of cases (range 0%–45%).[43] In an effort to minimize morbidity from unnecessary procedures, surgeons need to participate in the decisions surrounding staging, biopsy, or resection of lung nodules and provide guidance as to the best modality of tissue diagnosis or resection. With thoughtful input from surgeons and a multidisciplinary team, minimizing surgical intervention for benign disease without missing curable lung cancers is effective even in endemic areas with histoplasmosis.[45]

Future of Computed Tomography Screening

In the future, research studies and collaboration between surgical and nonsurgical organizations will refine the duration and frequency of CT screening for lung cancer as well as further define the high-risk populations that should be screened. Several new technological advances are expected to improve the efficiency and accuracy of CT screening programs. One of the most significant advancements will likely come with the development of computer software that will assist radiologists in more rapidly interpreting scans. Low-dose CT scans usually have 200 to 400 high-resolution sections that require on average 10 minutes for a radiologist to review compared with a breast mammogram, which averages 2 to 3 minutes per case.[46] Additional time savings may be realized if this technology can identify scans with no pulmonary nodules that would not, therefore, require formal interpretation by a thoracic radiologist. In addition to increased efficiency, it is anticipated that the software will also minimize the known variability in the interpretation of the scans as it relates to whether one or more nodules are present and have changed in appearance/volume compared with previous imaging.[42,47]

Other techniques are undergoing rigorous investigation and may prove to be valuable resources in screening for lung cancer in the future. Diagnostic biomarkers from blood or sputum[48] and other noninvasive specimens (eg, exhaled breath samples)[49] may also improve the accuracy of screening. Although no single biomarker or combination of biomarkers has yet been proven as effective in screening for and reducing mortality from lung cancer,[50] micro-RNAs and prosurfactant protein B show great promise.[51,52] From a surgical perspective, emerging technologies are also expected to refine and improve diagnostic and therapeutic techniques.[49] Advances in image-guided ablative therapies, such as radiation therapy, as well as targeted chemotherapy agents are also predicted to improve lung cancer survival.[8]

CRITERIA FOR DEVELOPING A HIGH-QUALITY COMPUTED TOMOGRAPHY SCREENING PROGRAM

Lung cancer screening should only be performed at institutions that have the appropriate infrastructure and expertise for the multidisciplinary workup of lung nodules and management of lung cancer. Screening programs need to be monitored and regulated by health care authorities in order to maintain appropriate standards of care. **Box 3** lists the minimal requirements and infrastructure for instituting a high-quality lung cancer screening program.[53–55] It is critical to remember that smoking cessation interventions must be an important component of a screening program as the cost-effectiveness of lung cancer screening improves between 20% and 45% when smoking cessation rates are achieved.[56]

Thoracic surgeons play a key role in the success of CT screening programs by providing expertise in the radiologic interpretation of lung nodules and recommendations for the appropriate diagnostic and therapeutic options available for surgical and nonsurgical patients. Furthermore, institutions considering the development of a lung cancer CT screening program need to ensure that they have access to a well–trained thoracic surgeon with experience in lung cancer management as well as a thoracic surgery unit with expertise in minimally invasive surgical techniques (eg, VATS) and comprehensive preoperative and postoperative care.

Box 3
Requirements for instituting a high-quality lung cancer screening program

- A coordinated referral network with centralized program coordination with structured reporting and patient data management system
- A dedicated and extensive continuing medical education program with effective communication strategy with outreach to patients, primary care, and referring physicians
- A chest imaging unit with low-dose high-resolution CT and PET imaging with expert thoracic radiologists able to provide standardized reporting of results
- An interventional radiology unit with expertise in percutaneous CT-guided needle biopsy techniques
- A respiratory medicine unit with expertise in pulmonary function testing, cardiopulmonary exercise testing, and pulmonary rehabilitation
- A pulmonary medicine unit with state-of-the-art video bronchoscopy equipment and expertise in bronchoscopic biopsy techniques, such as navigational bronchoscopy and EBUS
- A cytopathology department with expertise in lung cancer pathology and biomarkers as well as the ability to provide standardized reporting of results
- A thoracic surgery unit with expertise in minimally invasive surgical techniques
- Comprehensive preoperative and postoperative care unit
- A lung cancer–specific multidisciplinary tumor board
- An effective smoking cessation program with counseling
- Implementation of quality assurance measures to evaluate the performance of the program

Abbreviation: EBUS, endobronchial ultrasound.
  Data from Refs.[53–55]

SUMMARY

Despite the controversies in lung cancer screening, convincing evidence exists that low-dose CT screening of high-risk individuals decreases lung cancer mortality. To be effective and of high quality, screening programs need to be accessible to high-risk patients from all socioeconomic backgrounds, be performed in conjunction with a smoking cessation program, and have a communication strategy that focuses on educating patients and primary care physicians. Improvements in imaging techniques and efficiency of interpretation, diagnostic and therapeutic pathways, and surgical and nonsurgical techniques will also optimize the benefits of CT screening. Screening programs require input and coordinated participation from a multidisciplinary team including thoracic surgeons. Thoracic surgeons should be involved in the planning and implementation of a CT screening program and actively participate in the program in order to optimize the management of screen-detected lung nodules. Emerging technologies, such as molecular biomarkers, show promise for future screening modalities but require further validation.

ACKNOWLEDGMENTS

The authors would like to thank Ms Catherine MacPherson for her editorial assistance in the preparation of this article.

REFERENCES

1. Ferlay J, Soerjomataram I, Ervik M, et al. GLOBOCAN 2012 v1.0, Cancer incidence and mortality worldwide. IARC CancerBase No. 11 [Internet]. Lyon (France): International Agency for Research on Cancer; 2013. Available at: http://globocan.iarc.fr. Accessed July 15, 2014.
2. American Cancer Society. Cancer facts & figures 2014. Atlanta (GA): American Cancer Society; 2014. Available at: http://www.cancer.org/acs/groups/content/@research/documents/webcontent/acspc-042151.pdf. Accessed July 15, 2014.
3. Jemal A, Bray F, Center MM, et al. Global cancer statistics. CA Cancer J Clin 2011;61(2):69–90.
4. SEER 18 2004-2010, All races, both sexes by SEER summary stage 2000. Available at: http://seer.cancer.gov/statfacts/html/lungb.html. Accessed July 15, 2014.
5. Mausner JS, Kramer S. Screening in the detection of disease. In: Kramer S, editor. Epidemiology an

introductory text. 2nd edition. Philadelphia: W.B Saunders Company; 1985. p. 214–38.

6. Hennekens CH, Buring JE. Screening. In: Mayrent SL, editor. Epidemiology in medicine. 1st edition. Boston: Little, Brown and Company; 1987. p. 327–47.

7. Wilson JM, Jungner F. Principles and practice of screening for disease (Public Health Papers No. 34). Geneva (Switzerland): WHO; 1968. Available at: http://whqlibdoc.who.int/php/WHO_PHP_34.pdf. Accessed July 17, 2014.

8. Gill RR, Jaklitsch MT, Jacobson FL. Controversies in lung cancer screening. J Am Coll Radiol 2013; 10(12):931–6.

9. Oken MM, Hocking WG, Kvale PA, et al. Screening by chest radiograph and lung cancer mortality: the prostate, lung, colorectal, and ovarian (PLCO) randomized trial. JAMA 2011; 306(17):1865–73.

10. Detterbeck FC, Mazzone PJ, Naidich DP, et al. Screening for lung cancer: diagnosis and management of lung cancer, 3rd ed: American College of Chest Physicians evidence-based clinical practice guidelines. Chest 2013;143(5 Suppl):e78S–92S.

11. Doria-Rose VP, Marcus PM, Szabo E, et al. Randomized controlled trials of the efficacy of lung cancer screening by sputum cytology revisited. Cancer 2009;115(21):5007–17.

12. Melamed MR, Flehinger BJ, Zaman MB, et al. Screening for early lung cancer: results of the Memorial Sloan-Kettering Study in New York. Chest 1984;86(1):44–53.

13. Frost JK, Ball WC, Levin ML, et al. Early lung cancer detection: results of the initial (prevalence) radiologic and cytologic screening in the Johns Hopkins study. Am Rev Respir Dis 1984;130(4):549–54.

14. Fontana RS, Sanderson DR, Woolner LB, et al. Lung cancer screening; the Mayo program. J Occup Med 1986;28(8):746–50.

15. Manser R, Lethaby A, Irving LB, et al. Screening for lung cancer. Cochrane Database Syst Rev 2013;(6):CD001991.

16. Kubik A, Polak J. Lung cancer detection. Results of a randomized prospective study in Czechoslovakia. Cancer 1986;57(12):2427–37.

17. Marcus PM, Bergstralh EJ, Fagerstrom RM, et al. Lung cancer mortality in the Mayo lung project; impact of extended follow-up. J Natl Cancer Inst 2000;92(16):1308–16.

18. Wilde JA. 10 year follow-up of semi-annual screening for early detection of lung cancer in the Erfurt County, GDR. Eur Respir J 1989;2(7):656–62.

19. Gohagan JK, Marcus PM, Fagerstrom RM, et al, The Lung Screening Study Research Group. Final results of the Lung Screening Study, a randomized feasibility study of spiral CT versus chest x-ray screening for lung cancer. Lung Cancer 2005;47(1):9–15.

20. Infante M, Cavuto S, Lutman FR, et al. A randomized study of lung cancer screening with spiral computed tomography: three-year results from the DANTE trial. Am J Respir Crit Care Med 2009;180(5):445–53.

21. Aberle DR, Adams AM, Berg CD, et al. Reduced lung-cancer mortality with low-dose computed tomographic screening. N Engl J Med 2011; 365(5):395–409.

22. van den Bergh KA, Essink-Bot ML, Bunge EM, et al. Impact of computed tomography screening for lung cancer on participants in a randomized controlled trial (NELSON trial). Cancer 2008; 113(2):396–404.

23. Lopes Pegna A, Picozzi G, Mascalchi M, et al, ITALUNG Study Research Group. Design, recruitment and baseline results of the ITALUNG trial for lung cancer screening with low-dose CT. Lung Cancer 2009;64(1):34–40.

24. Saghir Z, Dirksen A, Ashraf H, et al. CT screening for lung cancer brings forward early disease. The randomized Danish Lung Cancer Screening Trial: status after five annual screening rounds with low-dose CT. Thorax 2012;67(4):296–301.

25. Pastorino U, Rossi M, Rosato V, et al. Annual or biennial CT screening versus observation in heavy smokers: 5-year results of the MILD trial. Eur J Cancer Prev 2012;21(3):308–15.

26. Becker N, Motsch E, Gross ML, et al. Randomized study on early detection of lung cancer with MSCT in Germany: study design and results of the first screening round. J Cancer Res Clin Oncol 2012; 138(9):1475–86.

27. Pastorino U. Current status of lung cancer screening. Thorac Surg Clin 2013;23(2):129–40.

28. Rocco G, Allen MS, Altorki NK, et al. Clinical statement on the role of the surgeon and surgical issues relating to computed tomography screening programs for lung cancer. Ann Thorac Surg 2013; 96(1):357–60.

29. Edwards JP, Datta I, Hunt JD, et al. The impact of computed tomographic screening for lung cancer on the thoracic surgery workforce. Ann Thorac Surg 2014;98(2):447–52. pii:S0003–4975(14)00862-5.

30. Jaklitsch MT, Jacobson FL, Austin JH, et al. The American Association for Thoracic Surgery guidelines for lung cancer screening using low-dose computed tomography scans for lung cancer survivors and other high-risk groups. J Thorac Cardiovasc Surg 2012;144(1):33–8.

31. NCCN guidelines version 2. 2014; lung cancer screening. Available at: http://www.nccn.org/professionals/physician_gls/pdf/lung_screening.pdf. Accessed July 20, 2014.

32. Field JK, Smith RA, Aberle DR, et al. International Association for the Study of Lung Cancer Computed Tomography Screening Workshop 2011 report. J Thorac Oncol 2012;7(1):10–9.

33. Wender R, Fontham ET, Barrera E Jr, et al. American Cancer Society lung cancer screening guidelines. CA Cancer J Clin 2013;63(2):107–17.

34. Roberts H, Walker-Dilks C, Sivjee K, et al. Screening high-risk populations for lung cancer: guideline recommendations. J Thorac Oncol 2013;8(10):1232–7.

35. Moyer VA, U.S. Preventative Services Task Force. Screening for lung cancer: U.S. Preventive Services Task Force recommendation statement. Ann Intern Med 2014;160(5):330–8.

36. Varlotto JM, Decamp MM, Flickinger JC, et al. Would screening for lung cancer benefit 75- to 84-year old residents of the United States? Front Oncol 2014;4:37.

37. McMahon PM, Meza R, Plevritis SK, et al. Comparing benefits from many possible computed tomography lung cancer screening programs: extrapolating from the National Lung Cancer Screening Trial using comparative modeling. PLoS One 2014;9(6):e99978.

38. De Koning H, Meza R, Plevritis SK, et al. Benefits and harms of computed tomography lung cancer screening strategies: a comparative modeling study for the U.S. Preventive Task Force. Ann Intern Med 2014;160(5):311–20.

39. McMahon H, Austin JH, Gamsu G, et al. Guidelines for the management of small pulmonary nodules detected on CT scans: a systematic review from the Fleischner Society. Radiology 2005;237(2):395–400.

40. Manos D, Seely JM, Taylor J, et al. The Lung Reporting and Data System (LU-RADS): a proposal for computed tomography screening. Can Assoc Radiol J 2014;65(2):121–34.

41. Jacobs PC, Gondrie MJ, van der Graaf Y, et al. Coronary artery calcium can predict all-cause mortality and cardiovascular events on low-dose CT screening for lung cancer. AJR AM J Roentgenol 2012;198(3):505–11.

42. Munden RF, Godoy MC. Lung cancer screening: state of the art. J Surg Oncol 2013;108(5):270–4.

43. Bach PB, Mirkin JN, Oliver TK, et al. Benefits and harms of CT screening for lung cancer: a systematic review. JAMA 2012;307(22):2418–29.

44. Flores R, Bauer T, Aye R, et al. Balancing curability and unnecessary surgery in the context of computed tomography screening for lung cancer. J Thorac Cardiovasc Surg 2014;147(5):1619–26.

45. Starnes RS, Reed MF, Meyer CA, et al. Can lung cancer screening by computed tomography be effective in areas with endemic histoplasmosis? J Thorac Cardiovasc Surg 2011;141:688–93.

46. Tammemagi MC, Lam S. Screening for lung cancer using low dose computed tomography. BMJ 2014; 348:g2253.

47. Armato SG 3rd, Roberts RY, Kocherginsky AM, et al. Assessment of radiologist performance in the detection of lung nodules: dependence on the definition of "truth". Acad Radiol 2009;16(1):28–38.

48. Gdowski A, Ranjan AP, Mukerjee A, et al. Nanobiosensors: role in cancer detection and diagnosis. Adv Exp Med Biol 2014;807:33–58.

49. Garg K, Hirsch FR, Kato Y, et al. Early detection and screening of lung cancer. Expert Rev Mol Diagn 2010;10(6):799–815.

50. Ghosal R, Kloer P, Lewis KE. A review of novel biological tools used in screening for the early detection of lung cancer. Postgrad Med J 2009; 85(1005):358–63.

51. Sozzi G, Boeri M, Rossi M, et al. Clinical utility of a plasma-based miRNA signature classifier within computed tomography lung cancer screening: a correlative MILD trial study. J Clin Oncol 2014; 32(8):768–73.

52. Sin DD, Tammemagi CM, Lam S, et al. Pro-surfactant protein B as a biomarker for lung cancer prediction. J Clin Oncol 2013;31(36):4536–43.

53. Frauenfelder T, Puhan MA, Lazor R, et al. Early detection of lung cancer: a statement from an expert panel of the Swiss university hospitals on lung cancer screening. Respiration 2014;87(3):254–64.

54. Mazzone P. The rationale for, and design of, a lung cancer screening program. Cleve Clin J Med 2012;79(5):337–45.

55. Arenberg D, Kazerooni EA. Setting up a lung cancer screening program. J Natl Compr Canc Netw 2012; 10(2):277–85.

56. Villanti AC, Jiang Y, Abrams DB, et al. A cost-utility analysis of lung cancer screening and the additional benefits of incorporating smoking cessation interventions. PLoS One 2013;8(8):e71379.

National Comprehensive Cancer Network (NCCN) Clinical Practice Guidelines for Lung Cancer Screening

Douglas E. Wood, MD

KEYWORDS

• Lung cancer • Screening • Low-dose computed tomography • Guidelines • Early detection

KEY POINTS

• Patients age 55 or older, with a smoking history of 30 pack-years or more, are eligible for lung cancer screening.
• Patients age 50 or older, with a smoking history of 20 pack-years or more, are eligible for lung cancer screening if they have an additional lung cancer risk factor (eg, asbestos exposure, chronic obstructive pulmonary disease, pulmonary fibrosis).
• Shared decision-making is important to make sure that patients are fully informed of benefits and risks of screening and that their personal preferences are the primary determinant of proceeding with lung cancer screening.
• An expert multidisciplinary team of thoracic radiologists, pulmonary physicians, and thoracic surgeons is important to evaluate and direct management of screen-detected lung nodules.
• Algorithmic management of screen-detected nodules is critically important to avoid the unintended harms of further diagnostic testing, invasive procedures, or surgery.

THE NATIONAL COMPREHENSIVE CANCER NETWORK

The National Comprehensive Cancer Network (NCCN) is a not-for-profit alliance of 25 of the world's leading cancer centers that are devoted to patient care, research, and education. The NCCN was created in 1995 as a national alliance to develop and institute standards of care for the treatment of cancer and perform outcomes research. The goal of the 13 original member institutions was to ensure delivery of high-quality, cost-effective services to people with cancer across the country. NCCN has become a developer and promoter of national programs to improve education, research, and patient care in oncology. Because the alliance has grown to 25 leading cancer centers, NCCN continues to concentrate on developing and communicating scientific and evaluative information to better inform the decision-making process between patients with cancer and their physicians.

NCCN is known particularly for their Clinical Practice Guidelines in Oncology and provides one of the most comprehensive and widely used set of cancer treatment guidelines in the United States and in the world (**Box 1**). In 2013,

The author has nothing to disclose.
Division of Cardiothoracic Surgery, Department of Surgery, University of Washington, 1959 Northeast Pacific, AA-115, Box 356310, Seattle, WA 98195-6310, USA
E-mail address: dewood@u.washington.edu

Thorac Surg Clin 25 (2015) 185–197
http://dx.doi.org/10.1016/j.thorsurg.2014.12.003
1547-4127/15/$ – see front matter © 2015 Elsevier Inc. All rights reserved.

NCCN.org reached a record high of more than 4.9 million PDF downloads of the NCCN Guidelines. However, less commonly known are areas of NCCN impact beyond the Clinical Practice Guidelines. The organization has now developed guidelines for patients that place the key principles of the physician guidelines into nontechnical language to empower patients and better inform them to be active participants in their cancer care. NCCN has also developed an oncology research program as well as the NCCN Foundation to improve the quality, effectiveness, and efficiency of care provided to patients with cancer. The organization has created a Drugs and Biologic Compendium (NCCN Compendium) and NCCN Chemotherapy Order Templates (NCCN Templates) as resources for cancer clinicians. NCCN.org provides free Web-based access to the clinical practice guidelines in all cancer areas to support providers in their decision-making in real-time practice settings. Finally, the alliance has established well-respected and robust educational programs that include specialty symposia and a more broadly based Annual Conference as well as focused Webinars on specific cancer topics that are widely used by cancer professionals around the world.

NATIONAL COMPREHENSIVE CANCER NETWORK GUIDELINES OVERVIEW

The NCCN Guidelines provide evidence-based and consensus-driven management that guides clinicians caring for patients with cancer. NCCN Guidelines are developed and updated by 47 individual panels that include more than 950 clinicians and oncology researchers from the 25 NCCN member institutions. These guidelines apply to more than 97% of patients living with cancer in the United States. Each panel consists of multidisciplinary, disease-specific subspecialists who are recognized experts in their field and provides a practical and pragmatic approach to cancer prevention, detection, and management. Each panel is assisted by high-level NCCN professional staff that analyzes and collates peer-reviewed research in the field, organizes complex management into straightforward algorithms, and helps to update the guidelines and the supporting article for each cancer site. A powerful strength of the guidelines is the incorporation of real-time updates in keeping with the rapid advancements in cancer research and management. The development of NCCN Guidelines is an ongoing and iterative process, based on a critical review of the best available evidence and recommendations by a multidisciplinary panel of experts in the field (**Box 2**).

The NCCN Guidelines Development Group comprises the NCCN Guidelines Steering Committee, panels specific to each of the guidelines, and the NCCN Headquarters Team that supports the panels and guideline activities. The steering committee provides oversight to the processes and planning of the NCCN Guidelines and oversees the institutional review process and implementation of NCCN Guidelines within their institutions. Each cancer or prevention site consists of an individual guideline panel led by a panel chair and vice chair. Each of the 25 member institutions nominates institutional representatives to the panel and the chair provides input into the selection of these representatives to ensure the inclusion and participation of relevant clinical expertise. The members of individual guidelines panels represent their institutions for all reviews and deliberations of the panel. Panel members actively participate in the evidence review, deliberations, and votes during the panel meetings and also present data relevant to agenda topics as assigned by the panel chair. The NCCN headquarters guidelines staff, comprising administrative support staff, editors, oncology scientists, and the senior NCCN leadership team, provide logistical and content support for all of the NCCN Guidelines and work in close collaboration with the panel to develop and update the algorithms and accompanying discussion section to reflect panel recommendations.

Transparency is an important principle of the NCCN Guidelines and the guidelines update process. The dates for all NCCN Guidelines panel meetings are posted and made publicly available on the NCCN Web site. In addition, important changes are also posted and made publicly available that capture the changes made to the recommendation category or indication and the addition or removal of drugs, and include a short summary of the panel discussion and rationale for the change.

An additional critical area of transparency is the management of conflicts of interests of panel members. Although the pharmaceutical and biotechnology industry plays a major role in cancer research and treatment, financial relationships with industry have the potential to introduce conflicts of interests and biases into the NCCN Guidelines process. NCCN has put in place a comprehensive policy for disclosure of financial relationships and for management of potential conflicts of interest. This policy mandates the disclosure of external financial relationships for all NCCN Guidelines panel members and recusal from deliberations of individuals with a meaningful conflict of interest. These policies are publicly available on the NCCN Web site and the full list of financial disclosures are posted and made publicly available relating to all members of the NCCN Guidelines panel, guidelines staff, and management team.

Although most cancer guidelines are updated only intermittently, NCCN Guidelines are reviewed and updated on a continuing basis to ensure that the recommendations are based on the most current evidence (**Box 3**). All active NCCN Guidelines are reviewed and updated at least annually. However, interim panel meetings are conducted throughout the year, as needed, based on new evidence that may change clinical practice standards. Issues or clinical questions relevant to the specific NCCN Guidelines are identified during the annual institutional review process and by external submission requests. New evidence in clinical data to support the annual panel deliberation is requested during the institutional review and external submission request processes and is also gathered from recent publications by the panel chair and NCCN headquarters guidelines staff. Although many changes relate to additional research, presentations, and experience in the field, some of the annual changes relate to clarification and improved application of the guidelines algorithm that relates to feedback or questions submitted to NCCN staff and the panel chair.

An important principle of NCCN Guidelines is the combination of evidence-based and consensus-based treatment algorithms. When high-level evidence is available, it is certainly the preferred data driving clinical decisions. However, in the real world, clinicians are often faced with important decisions for which there are only lower levels of scientific evidence or clinical experience

---

Box 3
National Comprehensive Cancer Network guideline update process

- Annual institutional review of guidelines
  - Solicitation by institutional panel representative for comments, updates, revisions
  - Directed to all related specialties/specialists at member institution
- Submission requests (external inquiries or data submissions)
- Panel meeting
  - Review of collated submissions and comments
  - Discussion, literature review, and voting on recommendations
- Updating of algorithm
- Review of algorithm by Panel Chair and Panel
- Further revision of algorithm
- Approval of updated algorithm by Panel Chair and Panel
- Posting of updated algorithm to NCCN Web site

on which to guide decision-making. In fact, most medical practice is based on relatively low levels of scientific evidence and based substantially on accrued knowledge from multiple nonrandomized studies, extrapolation from similar scientific studies as well as clinical experience that is passed down in training programs, medical meetings, and non-peer-reviewed publications. Different groups have recognized this variability in levels of evidence that support clinical guidelines and have published a variety of grading systems to characterize this evidence and the related recommendations. NCCN has provided a relatively simple grading used throughout all NCCN Guidelines. This list of categories of evidence and consensus is listed in **Box 4**. NCCN category 1 is used in the situation wherein there is high-level evidence that leads to uniform NCCN panel consensus regarding the intervention. However, the default evidence grade used throughout the NCCN Guidelines is category 2A, which represents uniform NCCN panel consensus, but is based on lower-level evidence. Category 2B recommendations are also based on lower-level evidence and where there is consensus, but not uniform consensus among the panel members. Category 3 recommendations represent those that are controversial, resulting in major NCCN panel member disagreement of whether the proposed intervention is appropriate or not.

DEVELOPMENT OF NEW GUIDELINES

Although the NCCN Guidelines have become comprehensive, covering virtually every aspect of cancer care, from time to time there is the identification of a new area of opportunity for guideline development. This is particularly true in the growing areas of cancer prevention, early cancer detection (screening), and end-of-life issues that relate to palliative and supportive care. The formal stepwise process of new guideline development is outlined in **Box 5**. The NCCN Guidelines Steering Committee identifies and selects a new topic to be addressed and, with the assistance of NCCN Guideline staff, selects a panel chair. The panel chair then works with NCCN staff to develop a matrix of relevant specialists and expertise to be represented on the panel as well as the initial development of literature to inform the evidence-based process. Each of the 25-member institutions is then solicited to nominate experts from their institution to serve on the panel.

Through an iterative process of teleconferences, Webinars, and face-to-face meetings, the panel develops an initial version of the guidelines that is reviewed, revised, and approved by the panel members. This initial version then goes through a second round of evaluation through institutional review at each of the 25-member institutions, leading to an additional round of revisions and improvements. The proposed draft and revisions are then collated and updated by the panel, leading to panel chair and panel approval and the posting and publication of the initial guidelines algorithm with supporting discussion and references.

DEVELOPMENT OF NATIONAL COMPREHENSIVE CANCER NETWORK GUIDELINES FOR LUNG CANCER SCREENING

Until 2010, Guidelines regarding lung cancer screening were incorporated within the NCCN Non-Small Cell Lung Cancer Panel (NSCL Panel) and included as a preface to the treatment guidelines for patients with NSCL. In fact, the 2010 guidelines from the NSCL Panel stated: "At the present time, the NCCN panel does not recommend the routine use of screening CT as standard clinical practice (category 3). Available data are

---

Box 4
National Comprehensive Cancer Network categories of evidence and consensus

- Category 1: based on high-level evidence, there is uniform NCCN consensus that the intervention is appropriate.
- Category 2A: based on lower-level evidence, there is uniform NCCN consensus that the intervention is appropriate.
- Category 2B: based on lower-level evidence, there is NCCN consensus that the intervention is appropriate.
- Category 3: based on any level of evidence, there is major NCCN disagreement that the intervention is appropriate.

All recommendations are category 2A unless otherwise noted.
From National Comprehensive Cancer Network. NCCN guidelines and clinical resources. Available at: http://www.nccn.org/professionals/physician_gls/categories_of_consensus.asp. Accessed November 26, 2014; with permission.

high-risk groups, risks of screening, benefits of screening, and accuracy of protocols and imaging modalities. A combination of workgroup meetings, Webinars, and face-to-face meetings led to preliminary drafts of the guidelines. However, the unexpected early release of the National Lung Screening Trial (NLST) results provided critical and important new information that substantively changed the evidence and the recommendations being considered by the panel. Major revisions of guidelines occurred after the November 2010 NLST results were released, leading to a preliminary draft version of the NCCN Guidelines for lung cancer screening in June 2011. A progressive period of panel and member institutional review further refined the draft guidelines, ultimately resulting in the final guidelines being published on October 26, 2011, the first major lung cancer screening guidelines to be developed following the publication of the NLST. Three annual revisions to the guidelines have been subsequently refined and published by the NCCN, the most recent being version 1.2015, published on July 22, 2014.

NATIONAL COMPREHENSIVE CANCER NETWORK GUIDELINES FOR LUNG CANCER SCREENING

The preface pages of the NCCN Guidelines list all of the individuals serving on the panel, their host institution, and their specialty. This page also includes a link to the conflict of interest disclosure for the panel members, followed by the table of contents that includes page links for navigating to relevant pages if one is using the electronic version of the guidelines from the Internet.

Risk Assessment and Inclusion Criteria

The first page of the NCCN Guidelines Lung Cancer Screening (LCS-1) is a risk assessment to identify and recommend a group of people in whom to recommend lung cancer screening (**Fig. 1**).[2] Relevant history includes smoking status (including extent, duration, and time from cessation), radon exposure, occupational exposure of agents known to increase lung cancer risk (eg, asbestos), cancer history (particularly other smoking-related cancers), disease history of chronic obstructive pulmonary disease (COPD) or pulmonary fibrosis, and secondhand smoke exposure. Patients are stratified into high risk, moderate risk, or low risk for the development of lung cancer (see **Fig. 1**). Patients stratified as high risk are considered eligible for screening and are recommended to undergo counseling and shared patient-physician decision-making that include a discussion of the benefits and risk of screening

conflicting and thus, conclusive data from ongoing clinical trials are necessary to define the benefits and risk."[1] However, increasing interest and publications relating to lung cancer screening led to a major part of the meeting devoted to this controversial topic by the NSCL Panel, yet without some of the key stakeholders and constituencies would provide the full breadth of information and expertise related to lung cancer screening.

At the 2009 annual update of the NCCN Guidelines for NSCL, the panel requested that the Guidelines Steering Committee consider establishment of a new panel dedicated to the topic of lung cancer screening. Later that same year, the Guidelines Steering Committee approved a new NCCN Guidelines for Lung Cancer Screening to be added to the existing guidelines on detection, prevention, and risk reduction for breast, prostate, cervical, and colorectal cancers. A timeline of the development of the NCCN Guidelines for Lung Cancer Screening is highlighted in **Box 6**. The panel was constituted in late 2009 and early 2010 and consisted of 26 specialists and experts representing thoracic radiology, pulmonary medicine, thoracic surgery, internal medicine, epidemiology, medical oncology, pathology, and a layperson representative.

To simplify and partition the guidelines development, 4 relevant workgroups were developed with corresponding workgroup chairs in the areas of

---

Box 6
Development of National Comprehensive Cancer Network guidelines for lung cancer screening (major events in bold)

- **October 2009: selection of chair for new guidelines panel for lung cancer screening.**
- **November 2009: nominations for panel members.**
- January 2010: literature search on lung cancer screening completed by oncology specialist and solicited from panel members.
- January 2010: first panel Web conference to discuss guidelines development process, disclosure requirements, panel membership, scope of guidelines, and panel assignments (4 workgroups)
  - High-risk groups
  - Risks of screening
  - Benefits of screening
  - Accuracy of protocols and imaging modalities
- March 2010: In-person panel meeting to discuss assignments and initiate guideline development.
- March to November 2010: ongoing development of evidence and guidelines through each of the 4 working groups.
- **November 2010: NLST results released.**
- November 2010: panel Web conference to discuss NLST results, follow-up on workgroup assignments, and refine evidence based on NLST results.
- May 2011: review of preliminary algorithm with panel chair.
- June 2011: preliminary draft version of NCCN Guidelines for lung cancer screening center panel for review.
- July 2011: panel Web conference to discuss comments received for the preliminary draft review and update guidelines.
- August 2011: preliminary draft version of the NCCN Guidelines for Lung Cancer Screening distributed for Institutional Review.
- September 2011: panel Web conference to discuss the institutional review comments.
- October 2011: updated version of guidelines sent to panel for final review.
- **October 2011: NCCN Guidelines for Lung Cancer Screening Version 1.2012 published at NCCN Web site (algorithm and discussion).**
- **June 2012: version 1.2013 published (algorithm and discussion).**
- **June 2013: version 1.2014 published (algorithm only).**
- April 2014: version 2.2014 published (updated discussion).
- **July 2014: version 1.2015 published (algorithm only).**

---

before embarking on an annual screening program with low-dose computed tomography (CT). Patients stratified to low or moderate risk are not recommended for routine lung cancer screening.

NCCN high-risk patients are stratified into 2 groups. The first group is analogous to the inclusion criteria of the NLST. This group is aged 55 to 74 years old with at least a 30 pack-year history of smoking, and if not a current smoker, has cessation of smoking period of less than 15 years. The NCCN panel graded this recommendation as a "Category 1" recommendation because of the high level of evidence from the NLST and uniform panel consensus. The second group contains patients with risk factors considered by the panel to be similar to the risk factors for NLST inclusion, as noted above, yet not evaluated within the context of a large randomized trial as was accomplished by the NLST. The panel considered the wide spectrum of evidence for lung cancer risk factors previously known and published to provide guidance to patients and their physicians as well as to avoid arbitrary exclusion of patients at high risk for developing lung cancer who had not been well-characterized by a randomized trial. This group of patients has frequently been nicknamed the "NCCN Group 2 patients." These patients are 50 years of age or older and have a

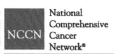

NCCN Guidelines Version 1.2015
Lung Cancer Screening

NCCN Guidelines Index
LCS Table of Contents
Discussion

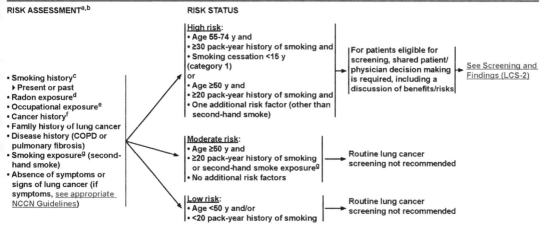

RISK ASSESSMENT[a,b]

RISK STATUS

• Smoking history[c]
  ‣ Present or past
• Radon exposure[d]
• Occupational exposure[e]
• Cancer history[f]
• Family history of lung cancer
• Disease history (COPD or pulmonary fibrosis)
• Smoking exposure[g] (second-hand smoke)
• Absence of symptoms or signs of lung cancer (if symptoms, see appropriate NCCN Guidelines)

High risk:
• Age 55-74 y and
• ≥30 pack-year history of smoking and
• Smoking cessation <15 y (category 1)
or
• Age ≥50 y and
• ≥20 pack-year history of smoking and
• One additional risk factor (other than second-hand smoke)

For patients eligible for screening, shared patient/physician decision making is required, including a discussion of benefits/risks → See Screening and Findings (LCS-2)

Moderate risk:
• Age ≥50 y and
• ≥20 pack-year history of smoking or second-hand smoke exposure[g]
• No additional risk factors

→ Routine lung cancer screening not recommended

Low risk:
• Age <50 y and/or
• <20 pack-year history of smoking

→ Routine lung cancer screening not recommended

[a]It is recommended that institutions performing lung cancer screening use a multidisciplinary approach that includes the specialties of thoracic radiology, pulmonary medicine, and thoracic surgery.
[b]Lung cancer screening is appropriate to consider for high-risk patients who are potential candidates for definitive treatment. Chest x-ray is not recommended for lung cancer screening.
[c]All current smokers should be advised to quit smoking, and former smokers should be advised to remain abstinent from smoking (http://www.surgeongeneral.gov/initiatives/tobacco/index.html). For additional cessation support and resources, smokers can be referred to http://www.smokefree.gov. Lung cancer screening should not be considered a substitute for smoking cessation.
[d]Documented high radon exposure.
[e]Agents that are identified specifically as carcinogens targeting the lungs: silica, cadmium, asbestos, arsenic, beryllium, chromium, diesel fumes, nickel, coal smoke, and soot.
[f]There is increased risk of developing new primary lung cancer among survivors of lung cancer, lymphomas, cancers of the head and neck, or smoking-related cancers.
[g]Individuals exposed to second-hand smoke have a highly variable exposure to the carcinogens, with varying evidence for increased risk after this variable exposure. Therefore, second-hand smoke is not independently considered a risk factor for lung cancer screening.

Note: All recommendations are category 2A unless otherwise indicated.
Clinical Trials: NCCN believes that the best management of any cancer patient is in a clinical trial. Participation in clinical trials is especially encouraged.

LCS-1

Fig. 1. NCCN LCS-1. (*Reproduced from* the NCCN Clinical Practice Guidelines in Oncology (NCCN Guidelines) for Lung Cancer Screening V.1.2015. © 2014 National Comprehensive Cancer Network, Inc. All rights reserved. The NCCN Guidelines and illustrations herein may not be reproduced in any form for any purpose without the express written permission of the NCCN. To view the most recent and complete version of the NCCN Guidelines, go online to NCCN.org. National Comprehensive Cancer Network, NCCN, NCCN Guidelines, and all other NCCN Content are trademarks owned by the National Comprehensive Cancer Network, Inc; with permission.)

20 pack-year or more smoking history, with at least one additional risk factor for smoking (other than secondhand smoke exposure). For example, a 67-year-old patient with a 25 pack-year smoking history, but also with occupational asbestos exposure, would be considered "high risk" within the NCCN group 2 criteria.

The inclusion of these NCCN group 2 patients into a high-risk group considered eligible for screening has been, perhaps, the most widely discussed and controversial aspect of the NCCN Guidelines. Extensive published data were provided within the article accompanying the guidelines that referenced each of these areas and their contribution to lung cancer risk.[2] The NCCN panel achieved consensus regarding the inclusion of this group as a high-risk category eligible for screening, yet at the lower, 2B level, because of a lack of uniformity among the panel members themselves. However, in the most recent iteration of the guidelines (version 1.2015), this recommendation

has been strengthened to a 2A recommendation representing uniform consensus of the NCCN panel.[3] Some guidelines from other groups that have been published subsequently have agreed with and endorsed these NCCN group 2 patients as being eligible for screening and have used the NCCN Guidelines as a template for their own recommendations,[4] whereas others have disagreed and have limited their recommendations for screening to those patients fulfilling only the NLST inclusion criteria.[5] The US Preventive Services Task Force (USPSTF) examined a variety of risk models in an effort to optimize recommendations for lung cancer screening.[6] The USPSTF recommendations also increased the age range to be considered eligible for screening, similar to the NCCN, but only evaluated the variables of age, smoking exposure, and duration of smoking cessation. Other known risk factors, such as asbestos exposure or underlying pulmonary fibrosis, were not evaluated in the USPSTF modeling study.

For patients deemed at high risk for lung cancer and therefore eligible for screening, a clear recommendation is made to invoke the process of "shared decision-making," encouraging an active dialogue between the physician and patient regarding the risks and benefits of lung cancer screening. Shared decision-making is a collaborative process that allows patients and their providers to make health care decisions together, taking into account the best scientific evidence available as well as the patient's values and preferences. Shared decision-making honors the patient's right to be fully informed of all care options and the potential harms and benefits. This process provides patients with the support they need to make the best individualized care decisions and is particularly important when it comes to preference-sensitive care, where there is more than one clinically appropriate treatment option, as there is in the case of screening. This process also allows the patient's values and preferences to be at the forefront of deciding whether to embark on screening for lung cancer.

Screening Interval and Duration

The second page of the NCCN Guidelines (LCS-2) directs the management of the initial findings on a baseline low-dose CT. When there is no lung nodules noted on the low-dose CT, the algorithm recommends continued low-dose CT for 2 years as a category 1 recommendation, or longer, until the patient is no longer eligible for definitive treatment, as a category 2A recommendation. Again, these differences in recommendations are on account of the high-level evidence provided by the NLST that only performed 2 years of follow-up CT scans. However, the NCCN, along with many others, has recognized that this level 1 evidence does not provide an adequate breadth of recommendation for patients and their providers who are embarking on lung cancer screening. Although the NLST demonstrated a 20% mortality benefit of 3 annual screens with low-dose CT, the view by most experts is that ongoing screening, as long as a patient is a candidate for treatment, is likely to provide additional mortality benefits. In fact, follow-up or "incidence" scans have a much higher yield of positive scans diagnosing early-stage lung cancer rather than being "false positives." This higher yield of positive scans is due to the historical baseline studies being available for comparison and therefore identifying truly new nodules that have a higher likelihood of malignancy. Ongoing follow-up scans also produce the paradoxic benefit of decreasing the false positive rate, with nodules that were initially deemed as

"positive" ultimately being recharacterized as "negative" because of persistent stability over time.

A second arm of the algorithm on this page acknowledges the possibility of detecting other abnormalities on the CT scan that may be unrelated to a potential diagnosis of lung cancer. There may be a suspicion of other malignancy, an identification of COPD or coronary artery calcifications, or other abnormalities that warrant additional investigation or referral to an appropriate specialist.

For patients that have detection of a lung nodule, the algorithm identifies 3 different scenarios: the identification of a solid or part solid nodule, the identification of a ground glass opacity (GGO) or nonsolid nodule, or the identification of multiple GGOs or nonsolid nodules. Each of these is directed to specific pages in the management guidelines.

Management of Screen Detected Nodules

One of the strengths of the NCCN Guidelines is the creation of clear algorithmic management of screen-detected nodules. Other guidelines have mostly concentrated on the identification of patients to be considered for screening. However, practitioners working in screening programs benefit from evidence-based guidance in the management of screen-detected abnormalities. Thoracic radiologists, pulmonary physicians, and thoracic surgeons work together in a multidisciplinary effort to evaluate nodules thoughtfully and efficiently. Although there is a strong imperative to detect early-stage lung cancer at a treatable stage, this must be balanced with an effort to minimize the unintended harms of additional diagnostic workup, invasive testing, and surgery. Nodule management algorithms help physicians make consistent and evidence-based recommendations in a way that can be explained and transparent to patients, cost-effective to society as well as defensible in a conservative risk-avoidance climate of medical decision-making. Multiple previous algorithms have been previously published that help direct nodule management. NCCN Guidelines have amalgamated published guidelines from the Fleischner society, International Early Lung Cancer Action Project (I–ELCAP), NLST, as well as European guidelines. In 2014, the American College of Radiology (ACR) published the Lung Imaging Reporting and Data System (LungRADS), a system designed to standardize lung cancer screening CT reporting and management recommendations, reduce confusion in lung cancer screening CT interpretations, and facilitate outcome monitoring. The

NCCN Lung Cancer Screening Panel and representatives from the ACR LungRADS project are currently working together to harmonize NCCN nodule management recommendations with LungRADS.

Page LCS-3 directs the further workup of solid or part solid nodules (**Fig. 2**). Nodules less than 6 mm are considered a "negative scan" and directed only to ongoing annual screening. A very important principle in any screening program is to try to minimize the unintended harms of screening by avoiding, to the degree possible, unnecessary additional diagnostic tests or invasive procedures. Data now exist from the I–ELCAP that shows minimal lost opportunity for identifying lung cancer, yet a substantial decrease in false positive findings by not initiating additional workup for nodules less than 6 mm.[7]

Nodules that are 6 to 8 mm are recommended to undergo a repeat low-dose CT in 3 months, and if stable, repeated at 6 months, and if continued stable, to revert to annual screening only. Nodules greater than 8 mm are to be considered for additional workup with PET. If the clinical, radiologic, and PET findings suggest a substantial suspicion of lung cancer, these patients are recommended for biopsy or surgical excision. On the other hand, if these lesions are a low suspicion for lung cancer, then they would be followed with a low-dose CT in 3 months, and if stable, a follow-up CT 6 months later, and if still stable, reverting to annual follow-up imaging.

The fourth page of the NCCN Guidelines (LCS-4) describes the nodule workup for GGO and nonsolid nodules, which are distinct from the workup of solid nodules (**Fig. 3**). Nodules 5 mm or less are followed simply with routine annual low-dose CT. However, if in follow-up, these have increased in size or have developed a solid or part solid component, then they would undergo either

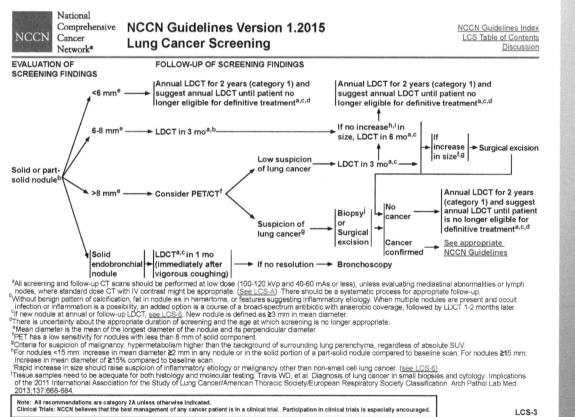

Fig. 2. NCCN LCS-3. IV, intravenous; LDCT, low-dose computed tomography; SUV, standard uptake value. (*Reproduced from* the NCCN Clinical Practice Guidelines in Oncology (NCCN Guidelines) for Lung Cancer Screening V.1.2015. © 2014 National Comprehensive Cancer Network, Inc. All rights reserved. The NCCN Guidelines and illustrations herein may not be reproduced in any form for any purpose without the express written permission of the NCCN. To view the most recent and complete version of the NCCN Guidelines, go online to NCCN.org. National Comprehensive Cancer Network, NCCN, NCCN Guidelines, and all other NCCN Content are trademarks owned by the National Comprehensive Cancer Network, Inc; with permission.)

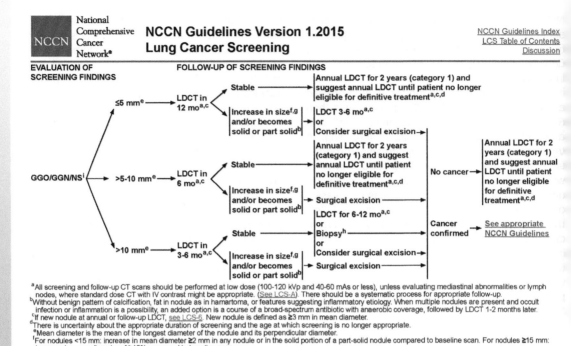

Fig. 3. NCCN LCS-4. GGN, ground glass nodule; IV, intravenous; NS, nonsolid. (*Reproduced from* the NCCN Clinical Practice Guidelines in Oncology (NCCN Guidelines) for Lung Cancer Screening V.1.2015. © 2014 National Comprehensive Cancer Network, Inc. All rights reserved. The NCCN Guidelines and illustrations herein may not be reproduced in any form for any purpose without the express written permission of the NCCN. To view the most recent and complete version of the NCCN Guidelines, go online to NCCN.org. National Comprehensive Cancer Network, NCCN, NCCN Guidelines, and all other NCCN Content are trademarks owned by the National Comprehensive Cancer Network, Inc; with permission.)

escalated interval follow-up low-dose CT in 3 to 6 months or consideration of surgical excision. Six-millimeter to 10-mm GGOs are recommended to undergo a follow-up low-dose CT in 6 months, and if stable, then revert to annual screening. If these nodules increase in size or become solid or part solid, then they are recommended to undergo surgical excision because of the high likelihood of adenocarcinoma or adenocarcinoma in situ. Nodules greater than 10 mm in size are recommended to undergo follow-up low-dose CT in 3 to 6 months. If they are stable, they have the option of undergoing continued radiologic surveillance at 6 to 12 months, biopsy, or surgical excision. Greater than 10-mm GGOs that increase in size or become solid or part solid are recommended to undergo surgical excision. The algorithms on both LCS-3 and LCS-4 direct the provider to the NCCN NSCL Panel Guidelines if lung cancer is identified.[8]

LCS-5 addresses the increasingly common scenario of multifocal GGOs and nonsolid nodules. For pure GGOs that are 5 mm or less, the recommendations are the same as for a single lesion, namely, annual surveillance low-dose CT only. Multifocal GGOs greater than 5 mm and without a dominant lesion are recommended to undergo a follow-up low-dose CT in 6 months and, if stable, will revert to annual screening. If these lesions increase in size or become part solid, the recommendation is analogous to those for a solitary lesion in recommending consideration of surgical excision. Multifocal disease with a dominant nodule with a part solid component is recommended to be followed sooner, with a low-dose CT in 3 to 6 months. If follow-up results in resolution, then these patients would return to annual low-dose CT, whereas if there is persistence or increase in the size of the dominant nodule, the algorithm directs back to the recommendations noted on LCS-3.

The sixth page of the NCCN Guidelines (LCS-6) addresses the identification of a new nodule found on annual or follow-up low-dose CT. Often these are related to a possible or probable inflammatory or infectious cause. If infection or inflammation is suspected based on clinical and radiologic characteristics, the guidelines recommend consideration of antimicrobials with a repeat low-dose CT in 1 to 2 months. Lesions that are resolved would revert to annual CT screening, whereas those that are resolving would be continued to be followed radiologically until resolution or stability is assured. Persistent or enlarging nodules would be further evaluated by PET and the algorithms already described on LCS-3 and LCS-4 followed. If infection or inflammation is not suspected based on radiologic or clinical findings, then these patients would be managed according to the relevant preceding nodule management algorithms (LCS-3, LCS-4, or LCS-5).

Additional Materials

Page LCS-A of the guidelines provided tables that provide guidance regarding the acquisition, storage, interpretation, and nodule reporting for low-dose CT. This page provides benchmarks and guidance for radiation exposure, and details of image acquisition protocols. It also provides recommendations regarding interpretation tools and recommended definitions for reporting of clinically important nodule parameters.

Page LCS-B lists the known and projected risks and benefits of lung cancer screening. Although this list is not necessarily comprehensive, it is meant to outline the major potential risks of embarking on lung cancer screening as well as the potential benefits of screening that is highlighted by the decrease in lung cancer mortality; this is meant to provide further information for patients and their health care providers to inform the shared decision-making that is important for individualized patient choice and preferences regarding lung cancer screening.

Finally, the algorithm is supported by an extensive discussion, which is a 27-page article with 287 references that provides the rationale and documentation behind the guidelines. The discussion provides the rationale and references for the identification of high-risk individuals, the accuracy of low-dose CT protocols as well as the benefits and risks of lung cancer screening. Along with the algorithm, this discussion is updated annually to remain current and to add and refine new and relevant references.

UPDATE TO NATIONAL COMPREHENSIVE CANCER NETWORK GUIDELINES FOR LUNG CANCER SCREENING V.1.2013

A major weakness of nearly all guidelines is the static nature of the recommendations in a field of constantly changing data and advances in practice. In rapidly changing areas of medicine, guidelines may even be outdated by the time they are published. A major strength of the NCCN Guidelines is the commitment to continual revisions and updates to keep the guidelines current, relevant, and meaningful to health care providers and their patients. NCCN Guidelines are updated at least annually through a robust process of individual and institutional suggestions for revision, and a thorough evidence-based and consensus-based update process that is as thoroughly scrutinized as the original guidelines. If important new data are presented or published that would direct significant guideline changes, the NCCN panel can be convened in between annual updates to address specific new topics or recommendations as they arise. In practice, these updates not only keep the guidelines fresh and topical with current data but also use feedback from users to improve and clarify areas of confusion or unclear recommendations.

The first NCCN Guidelines for Lung Cancer Screening update was published in June 2012. The most significant change in this update was a revision of the recommendations regarding screening intervals. The initial baseline scan with 2 annual low-dose CTs was clarified as a category 1 recommendation, but language was added to "consider annual low-dose computed tomography (LDCT) until patient no longer eligible for definitive treatment," rather than the previous recommendation to screen until age 74 (derived from the NLST). This recommendation acknowledged the somewhat arbitrary age boundary and limits of a clinical trial application to actual clinical practice, and the fact that as long as patients were eligible for treatment that they should still be candidates for screening. Several other minor changes were made for better refinement and clarification, including footnotes on LCS-1 that helped define the multidisciplinary lung cancer screening team, emphasizing the importance of smoking cessation counseling, and refined the list of agents that are identified as carcinogens targeting the lungs. Page LCS-2 was newly created and broken off from LCS-1 to improve the algorithm clarity in the management of screen-detected findings. Additional minor revisions included recommendations about the interpretation of PET findings and the management of suspected infection or inflammation detected on annual low-dose CT screening.

UPDATE TO NATIONAL COMPREHENSIVE CANCER NETWORK GUIDELINES FOR LUNG CANCER SCREENING V.1.2014

The second NCCN Guidelines Lung Cancer Screening revision was published in June 2013 with additional revisions in the Discussion published as a further update in April 2014. There were 2 substantive changes in this update of the guidelines. The first was a change in the size criteria to define a "positive" scan. The original guidelines had recommended further evaluation with shorter interval low-dose CT for lung nodules greater than 4 mm. New data had been published by Henschke and colleagues[7] in the I–ELCAP lung cancer screening experience that demonstrated no loss in diagnostic sensitivity yet far fewer follow-up diagnostic studies if 6 mm was used to define a "positive" scan rather than 4 mm. Therefore, the algorithm on page LCS-3 was revised to eliminate evaluation of 4-mm to 6-mm nodules; both respond to this important new data as well as to improve the guidelines by decreasing further diagnostic studies of patients with very small nodules.

The second major change was the addition of a new page, LCS-5, to address the evaluation and management of multiple GGOs and nonsolid lesions. This change was recognized by the panel as an increasingly frequent clinical scenario that would benefit from additional guidance in the guidelines.

Several other minor revisions were incorporated in footnotes that recommended against chest radiograph for lung cancer screening, a further emphasis on smoking cessation, and clarification about the need for a systematic process for appropriate follow-up of screen-detected findings.

UPDATE TO NATIONAL COMPREHENSIVE CANCER NETWORK GUIDELINES FOR LUNG CANCER SCREENING V.1.2015

The third revision of the NCCN Guidelines Lung Cancer Screening was published in July 2014 with the most significant change being an upgrade of recommendations for screening in NCCN group 2 patients from a 2B recommendation to a 2A recommendation. Although this group of patients had remained one of the most controversial areas of NCCN Guidelines, the panel expressed uniform consensus of the appropriateness these patients being eligible for lung cancer screening. However, the panel also added important language about shared patient-physician decision-making to be part of informing patients eligible for lung cancer screening about the benefits and risks, and helping to make individualized choices that empower patients to select or defer lung cancer screening based on their own personal preferences and beliefs. A second significant change was a recommendation of a preference for a 1-mm or less slice width on low-dose CT imaging. To help clarify the technical aspects of CT acquisition, storage, interpretation, and nodule reporting, a new table was added to the guidelines addressing these low-dose CT details. Recommendations were also added for standardized reporting of lung nodules, such as LungRADS developed by the ACR and other minor footnote updates.

SUMMARY

The NCCN represents 25 major cancer centers in the United States and has a wide breadth of experience in the development of cancer treatment guidelines. Through a rigorous and transparent process that includes multidisciplinary expert panels from all 25 institutions, NCCN produces guidelines in cancer prevention and early detection as well as cancer management that cover nearly all malignant conditions. In 2009, the NCCN created a new Lung Cancer Screening Panel that had the benefit of the publication of the NLST results during the guidelines development. This large prospective randomized trial that demonstrated a 20% mortality benefit from low-dose CT screening for lung cancer shaped the NCCN Guidelines and subsequent guidelines published by other organizations. The NCCN Lung Cancer Screening Panel amalgamated data from the NLST as well as other preceding literature on lung cancer risk factors to develop recommendations of patients who should be eligible for lung cancer screening. These risk factors consist of patients analogous to those included in the NLST (ie, age 55–74 and at least 30 pack-year smoking history). However, NCCN also characterized a second group (NCCN group 2) as having a similar risk profile to be considered eligible for screening. These patients are aged 50 or older, with 20 pack-year or more smoking history, with at least one additional lung cancer risk factor. The NCCN Guidelines for Lung Cancer Screening provide algorithmic recommendations for the management of screen-detected nodules that cover nearly all clinical scenarios faced by physicians in screening programs. The guidelines are practical, evidence-based, and consensus-based and are updated annually to maintain currency with newly published data and relevance to physicians and their patients. Shared decision-making with physicians and patients is an important principle to follow before embarking on an elective process of cancer screening whereby harms must be carefully balanced against the benefits of screening.

REFERENCES

1. Ettinger DS, Akerley W, Bepler G, et al. Non-small cell lung cancer. J Natl Compr Canc Netw 2010; 8(7):740 801.
2. Wood DE, Eapen GA, Ettinger DS, et al. Lung cancer screening. J Natl Compr Canc Netw 2012;10:24–65.
3. Referenced with permission from the NCCN Clinical Practice Guidelines in Oncology (NCCN Guidelines®) for Lung Cancer Screening V.1.2015. © National Comprehensive Cancer Network, Inc 2014. All rights reserved. Accessed [September 12, 2014]. To view the most recent and complete version of the guideline, go online to NCCN.org. National Comprehensive Cancer Network®, NCCN®, NCCN Guidelines®, and all other NCCN Content are trademarks owned by the National Comprehensive Cancer Network, Inc.
4. Jaklistch MT, Jacobson FL, Austin JH, et al. The American Association for Thoracic Surgery guidelines for lung cancer screening using low-dose computed tomography scans for lung cancer survivors and other high risk groups. J Thorac Cardiovasc Surg 2012;144:33–8.
5. Bach PB, Mirkin JN, Oliver TK, et al. Benefits and harms of CT screening for lung cancer: a systematic review. JAMA 2012;307:2418–29.
6. De Koning HJ, Meza R, Plevritis SK, et al. Benefits and harms of computed tomography lung cancer screening strategies: a comparative modeling study for the US Preventive Services Task Force. Ann Intern Med 2014;160:311–20.
7. Henschke CI, Yip R, Yankelevitz DF, et al, International Early Lung Cancer Action Project Investigators. Definition of a positive result in computed tomography screening for lung cancer. Ann Intern Med 2013;148:246–52.
8. Ettinger DS, Akerley W, Borghaei H, et al. Non-small cell lung cancer, version 2.2013. J Natl Compr Canc Netw 2013;11:645–53.

The United States Preventive Services Task Force Recommendations for Lung Cancer Screening

CrossMark

Shanda H. Blackmon, MD, MPH[a],*,
Shamiram R. Feinglass, MD, MPH[b]

KEYWORDS

- United States Preventive Services Task Force • Lung cancer screening
- Agency for Healthcare Research and Quality • Computed tomography scanning • Lung cancer

KEY POINTS

- The United States Preventive Services Task Force was created in 1984 and conducts scientific evidence reviews of a broad range of clinical preventive health care services.
- The United States Preventive Services Task Force is supported by the Agency for Healthcare Research and Quality.
- In 2013, the United States Preventive Services Task Force made a grade B recommendation for annual screening for lung cancer with low-dose computed tomography in adult patients age 55 to 80 years who have a 30 pack-year smoking history and currently smoke or have quit within the last 15 years.
- There is currently an open National Coverage Analysis for low-dose computed tomography screening for lung cancer.

WHAT IS THE UNITED STATES PREVENTIVE SERVICES TASK FORCE?

Created in 1984, the United States Preventive Services Task Force (USPSTF) is an independent, volunteer panel of 16 nonfederal national expert members in evidence-based medicine, prevention, or primary care, which may include family physicians, behavioral health specialists, epidemiologists, internists, pediatricians, or nurses. The panel is led by a chair and 2 vice chairs. Task Force members are appointed by the Director of Agency for Healthcare Research and Quality (AHRQ) to serve 4-year volunteer terms. Members are screened to ensure that they have no substantial conflicts of interest that could impair the scientific integrity of the Task Force's work. They conduct scientific evidence reviews of a broad range of clinical preventive health care services (such as screening, counseling, and preventive medications) and develop recommendations for primary care clinicians and health systems. Coverage, policy, or implementation strategies are beyond the scope of the USPSTF. Within the recommendations are clinician-oriented and patient-oriented fact sheets. These recommendations are published in the form of Recommendation Statements.

The recommendations of USPSTF are based on a review of existing peer-reviewed evidence and

Disclosure: The authors have nothing to disclose; no financial relationships, paid speaker fees, or any other relationship with a commercial company that has a direct financial interest in the subject matter.
[a] Thoracic Surgery, Mayo Clinic, 200 First Street, Southwest, Rochester, MN 55905, USA; [b] The Feinglass Group, 1604 S. Woodfield Trail, Warsaw, IN 46580, USA
* Corresponding author.
E-mail address: blackmon.shanda@mayo.edu

are intended to help primary care clinicians and patients decide together whether a preventive service is right for a patient's needs. The Task Force assigns each recommendation a letter grade (A, B, C, or D grade or an "I" statement) based on the strength of the evidence and the balance of benefits and harms of a preventive service (**Table 1**). The recommendations apply only to people who have no signs or symptoms of the specific disease or condition under evaluation, and the recommendations address only services offered in the primary care setting or services referred by a primary care clinician.

Since 1998, the AHRQ has been authorized by the US Congress to convene the Task Force and to provide ongoing scientific, administrative, and dissemination support to the Task Force. AHRQ originally began as the Agency for Health Care Policy and Research and was tasked with producing guidelines and is one of 12 agencies within the United States Department of Health and Human Services.[1]

Each year, the Task Force reports to Congress critical evidence gaps in research related to clinical preventive services and recommends priority areas that deserve further examination. **Fig. 1** shows how the USPSTF plays a role in coverage in the United States.

HOW HAS THE UNITED STATES PREVENTIVE SERVICES TASK FORCE PLAYED A ROLE IN THE COVERAGE PROCESS FOR LUNG CANCER SCREENING?

In 2013, the USPSTF made a grade B recommendation for annual screening for lung cancer with LDCT in adult patients age 55 to 80 years who have a 30 pack-year smoking history and currently smoke or have quit within the last 15 years. They deemed screening unnecessary once a person has not smoked for 15 years or develops a health problem that substantially limits life expectancy or the ability or willingness to have curative lung surgery.[2]

WHAT WERE THE SPECIFIC THE UNITED STATES PREVENTIVE SERVICES TASK FORCE RECOMMENDATIONS?

The USPSTF found adequate evidence that annual screening for lung cancer with LDCT in a defined population of high-risk persons can prevent a

Table 1
Grade of USPSTF recommendation

Grade	Definition	Suggestions for Practice
A	The USPSTF recommends the service. There is high certainty that the net benefit is substantial.	Offer or provide this service.
B	The USPSTF recommends the service. There is high certainty that the net benefit is moderate or there is moderate certainty that the net benefit is moderate to substantial.	Offer or provide this service.
C	The USPSTF recommends selectively offering or providing this service to individual patients based on professional judgment and patient preferences. There is at least moderate certainty that the net benefit is small.	Offer or provide this service for selected patients depending on individual circumstances.
D	The USPSTF recommends against the service. There is moderate or high certainty that the service has no net benefit or that the harms outweigh the benefits.	Discourage the use of this service.
I Statement	The USPSTF concludes that the current evidence is insufficient to assess the balance of benefits and harms of the service. Evidence is lacking, of poor quality, or conflicting, and the balance of benefits and harms cannot be determined.	Read the clinical considerations section of USPSTF Recommendation Statement. If the service is offered, patients should understand the uncertainty about the balance of benefits and harms.

From U.S. Preventative Service Task Force. Grade Definitions after July 2012. What the grades mean and suggestions for practice. Available at: http://www.uspreventiveservicestaskforce.org/Page/Name/grade-definitions#grade-definitions-after-july-2012. Accessed November 21, 2014.

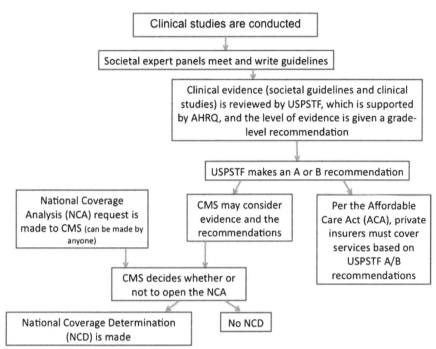

Fig. 1. USPSTF coverage role in the United States as of 2014. (*Adapted from* U.S. Preventative Services Task Force. Procedure manual. AHRQ publication no. 08-05118-EF. 2008. Available at: http://www.uspreventiveservicestask-force.org/Page/Name/procedure-manual. Accessed December 3, 2014.)

substantial number of lung cancer–related deaths. Direct evidence from the National Lung Screening Trial (NLST), which was a large, well-conducted, randomized, controlled trial, provided moderate certainty of the benefit of lung cancer screening with LDCT in this population.[3] They noted screening cannot prevent most lung cancer–related deaths, and smoking cessation remains essential.

The USPSTF found insufficient evidence on the harms associated with incidental findings. Overdiagnosis of lung cancer occurs, but its precise magnitude is uncertain. A modeling study performed for the USPSTF estimated that 10% to 12% of screen-detected cancer cases are overdiagnosed—that is, they would not have been detected in the patient's lifetime without screening.[2] Radiation harms, including cancer resulting from cumulative exposure to radiation, vary depending on the age at the start of screening, the number of scans received, and the person's exposure to other sources of radiation, particularly other medical imaging.

The USPSTF concluded with moderate certainty that annual screening for lung cancer with LDCT is of moderate net benefit in asymptomatic persons who are at high risk for lung cancer based on age, total cumulative exposure to tobacco smoke, and years since quitting smoking. The

moderate net benefit of screening depends on limiting screening to persons who are at high risk, the accuracy of image interpretation being similar to that found in the NLST, and the resolution of most false-positive results without invasive procedures.[3] The USPSTF recommended extending the program used in the NLST through age 80 years. The USPSTF recommended discontinuing screening if a person has not smoked for 15 years or if the person develops a health problem that substantially limits life expectancy or the ability or willingness to have curative lung surgery. USPSTF determined current evidence was lacking on the net benefit of expanding LDCT screening to include lower-risk patients.[2] USPSTF supports the future development of risk assessment tools to help clinicians better individualize patients' risks.[4]

SMOKING CESSATION COUNSELING

To be consistent with the USPSTF recommendation on counseling and interventions to prevent tobacco use and tobacco-caused disease, persons who are referred to a lung cancer screening program through primary care should receive smoking cessation interventions before referral. Because many persons may enter screening through pathways besides referral from primary care, the USPSTF encouraged incorporating such interventions into the screening program.

OTHER UNITED STATES PREVENTIVE SERVICES TASK FORCE RECOMMENDATIONS RELATED TO LUNG CANCER SCREENING

Shared decision making is a part of the framework of every USPSTF recommendation and is emphasized in their recommendations for lung cancer screening. The USPSTF supports adherence to quality standards for LDCT[5] and establishing protocols to follow up on abnormal results, such as those standards proposed by the National Comprehensive Cancer Network.[6] The Network recommended mechanisms be implemented to ensure adherence to these standards. The USPSTF encourages the development of a registry to ensure that appropriate data are collected from screening programs to foster continuous improvement over time. The registry should also compile data on incidental findings and the testing and interventions that occur as a result of these findings. This recommendation was made to help future analyses clarify issues related to the management of indeterminate nodules. Several studies were used in the USPSTF recommendation process.[3,7–19] These studies specifically aided them in determining the effectiveness of early detection and treatment, estimating the magnitude of net benefit and determining how the evidence fits with biologic understanding. The USPSTF did not cite the American Association of Thoracic Surgeons Guidelines or the American College of Surgeons Guidelines for lung cancer screening as part of this section analyzed, but do refer to their findings as sources.[20,21]

OPENING THE UNITED STATES PREVENTIVE SERVICES TASK FORCE RECOMMENDATION TO PUBLIC COMMENT

A draft version of the recommendation statement was posted for public comment on the USPSTF Web site from 30 July to 26 August 2013. In response to comments, the USPSTF further emphasized the importance of tobacco cessation as the primary way to prevent lung cancer and provided links to resources that clinicians can use to help their patients quit smoking. A section on implementation of a screening program was added, emphasizing the need for monitoring this implementation, quality assurance in diagnostic imaging, and appropriate follow-up to replicate the benefits observed in the NLST in the general population. The USPSTF also clarified that, in addition to age and smoking history, such risk factors as occupational exposure, family history, and history of other lung diseases are important when assessing patients' risks for lung cancer.

The USPSTF acknowledged the importance of accurately identifying persons who are at highest risk to maximize the benefits and minimize the harms of screening and calls for more research to improve risk assessment tools. The USPSTF did not incorporate the costs of a screening program or the potential savings from a reduction in treatment of advanced lung cancer into the recommendation.

UPDATE OF PREVIOUS UNITED STATES PREVENTIVE SERVICES TASK FORCE RECOMMENDATION

This recommendation updates the 2004 recommendation, in which the USPSTF concluded that the evidence was insufficient to recommend for or against screening for lung cancer in asymptomatic persons with LDCT, chest radiography, sputum cytologic evaluation, or a combination of these tests. Currently, the USPSTF recommends annual screening for lung cancer with LDCT in persons who are at high risk based on age and cumulative tobacco smoke exposure.

WHAT DOES UNITED STATES PREVENTIVE SERVICES TASK FORCE RECOMMENDATION MEAN FOR MEDICARE BENEFICIARIES?

There is currently an open National Coverage Analysis for LDCT screening for lung cancer, which was scheduled to be issued November of 2014. As part of this process, a Medicare Evidence Development and Coverage Advisory Committee was convened at the request of the Centers for Medicare and Medicaid to assist in reviewing evidence. The committee met April 30, 2014. When answering the question, "How confident are you that there is adequate evidence to determine if the benefits outweigh the harms of lung cancer screening with LDCT... in the Medicare population?" the committee found low confidence in LDCT for screening.[22]

HOW WILL UNITED STATES PREVENTIVE SERVICES TASK FORCE RECOMMENDATIONS AFFECT PRIVATE INSURERS?

In practical terms, the USPSTF recommendations will likely mean a large increase in actual screening rates. Primary care physicians largely had not been recommending computed tomography lung cancer screening, which few insurance companies previously covered. Under the Affordable Care Act, insurance companies are now required to cover any screening service that is given an A or

B rating by the USPSTF without any copay or deductible.

REFERENCES

1. Healthcare Research and Quality Act of 1999. Available at: http://www.ahrq.gov/policymakers/hrqa99a.html. Accessed August 8, 2014.
2. USPSTF website. Available at: http://www.uspreventiveservicestaskforce.org/uspstf/uspslung.htm. Accessed August 8, 2014.
3. Aberle DR, Adams AM, Berg CD, et al, National Lung Screening Trial Research Team. Reduced lung-cancer mortality with low-dose computed tomographic screening. N Engl J Med 2011; 365(5):395–409.
4. Kovalchik SA, Tammemagi M, Berg CD, et al. Targeting of low-dose CT screening according to the risk of lung-cancer death. N Engl J Med 2013;369(3): 245–54.
5. Medicare Improvements for Patients and Providers Act. 2008. 42 U.S.C. §101-304.
6. National Comprehensive Cancer Network. National Comprehensive Cancer Network clinical practice guidelines in oncology: lung cancer screening. Fort Washington (PA): National Comprehensive Cancer Network; 2014.
7. Humphrey L, Deffebach M, Pappas M, et al. Screening for lung cancer: systematic review to update the U.S. Preventive Services Task Force Recommendation Statement. Evidence synthesis no. 105. AHRQ publication no. 13-05196-EF-1. Rockville (MD): Agency for Healthcare Research and Quality; 2013.
8. Humphrey LL, Deffebach M, Pappas M, et al. Screening for lung cancer with low-dose computed tomography: a systematic review to update the U.S. Preventive Services Task Force recommendation. Ann Intern Med 2013;159:411–20.
9. de Koning HJ, Plevritis S, Hazelton WD, et al. Benefits and harms of computed tomography lung cancer screening programs for high-risk populations. AHRQ publication no. 13-05196-EF-2. Rockville (MD): Agency for Healthcare Research and Quality; 2013.
10. de Koning HJ, Meza R, Plevritis SK, et al. Benefits and harms of lung cancer screening: modeling strategies for the U.S. Preventive Services Task Force. Ann Intern Med 2014;160(5):311–20.
11. Church TR, Black WC, Aberle DR, et al, National Lung Screening Trial Research Team. Results of initial low-dose computed tomographic screening for lung cancer. N Engl J Med 2013;368(21): 1980–91.
12. Pinsky PF, Church TR, Izmirlian G, et al. The national lung screening trial: results stratified by demographics, smoking history, and lung cancer histology. Cancer 2013;119(22):3976–83.
13. Infante M, Lutman FR, Cavuto S, et al, DANTE Study Group. Lung cancer screening with spiral CT: baseline results of the randomized DANTE trial. Lung Cancer 2008;59(3):355–63.
14. Infante M, Cavuto S, Lutman FR, et al, DANTE Study Group. A randomized study of lung cancer screening with spiral computed tomography: three-year results from the DANTE trial. Am J Respir Crit Care Med 2009;180(5):445–53.
15. Saghir Z, Dirksen A, Ashraf H, et al. CT screening for lung cancer brings forward early disease. The randomised Danish Lung Cancer Screening Trial: status after five annual screening rounds with low-dose CT. Thorax 2012;67(4):296–301.
16. Pastorino U, Rossi M, Rosato V, et al. Annual or biennial CT screening versus observation in heavy smokers: 5-year results of the MILD trial. Eur J Cancer Prev 2012;21(3):308–15.
17. Oken MM, Hocking WG, Kvale PA, et al, PLCO Project Team. Screening by chest radiograph and lung cancer mortality: the Prostate, Lung, Colorectal, and Ovarian (PLCO) randomized trial. JAMA 2011; 306(17):1865–73.
18. Veronesi G, Maisonneuve P, Bellomi M, et al. Estimating overdiagnosis in low-dose computed tomography screening for lung cancer: a cohort study. Ann Intern Med 2012;157(11):776–84.
19. Bach PB, Mirkin JN, Oliver TK, et al. Benefits and harms of CT screening for lung cancer: a systematic review. JAMA 2012;307(22):2418–29.
20. Jaklitsch MT, Jacobson FL, Austin JH, et al. The American Association for Thoracic Surgery guidelines for lung cancer screening using low-dose computed tomography scans for lung cancer survivors and other high-risk groups. J Thorac Cardiovasc Surg 2012;144(1):33–8.
21. Wender R, Fontham ET, Barrera E Jr, et al. American Cancer Society lung cancer screening guidelines. CA Cancer J Clin 2013;63(2):107–17.
22. Available at: http://www.cms.gov/medicare-coverage-database/details/medcac-meeting-details.aspx?MEDCACId=68. Accessed August 8, 2014.

Current Estimate of Costs of Lung Cancer Screening in the United States

David C. Mauchley, MD, John D. Mitchell, MD*

KEYWORDS

- Lung cancer screening ● Low-dose computed tomography (LDCT) ● Cost-effectiveness
- National Lung Screening Trial (NLST) ● Early Lung Cancer Action Project (ELCAP)
- Budget impact model

KEY POINTS

- The results of the National Lung Screening Trial indicate that some lung cancer deaths can be prevented with low-dose computed tomography (LDCT) screening in a high-risk population.
- Based on current calculations, the cost of screening high-risk patients for lung cancer with LDCT is comparable with that of screening for colon cancer and breast cancer.
- With improving computed tomography scan technology and implementation of smoking cessation, the cost of LDCT screening could be further reduced.

INTRODUCTION

Before publication of the results of the National Lung Screening Trial (NLST) in 2011, there was only a theoretic benefit to screening patients at high risk for developing lung cancer with low-dose helical computed tomography (LDCT). This trial was stopped early when data showed a 20% reduction in lung cancer mortality in the LDCT arm compared with the chest radiograph (CXR) arm.[1] These findings have led to the support of multiple organizations and societies for screening high-risk patients with LDCT. Notably, the US Preventive Services Task Force (USPTF) now recommends screening for patients aged 55 to 80 years who are current smokers (or recently quit) with a 30-pack-year smoking history. This recommendation is classified as B grade by the USPTF, which positions lung cancer with other malignancies such as cervical, breast, and colon for which there are objective data supporting dissemination of screening on a national level.[2]

Despite the data from NLST and the recommendation from the USPTF, there is still considerable controversy surrounding the implementation of LDCT screening on a national level. Individuals opposed to widespread screening argue that the false-positive rate in screened patients (estimated as 96.4% in NLST) leads to a significant number of unnecessary imaging tests and procedures as well as psychological distress for the patients. There is also concern that the financial burden imposed on the United States health care system by the additional scans and associated follow-up tests would overwhelm the benefit achieved by the reduction in mortality. There have been several studies evaluating the cost-effectiveness of screening for lung cancer with LDCT. This article summarizes previous efforts at estimating the cost of LDCT screening for lung cancer, provides an up-to-date estimation of the annual cost in the United States if the practice of widespread screening were adopted, identifies factors that have the greatest effect on cost, and reviews future issues

Disclosure: The authors report no conflicts of interest regarding the content of this article.
Division of Cardiothoracic Surgery, University of Colorado School of Medicine, 12631 East 17th Avenue, C-310, Aurora, CO 80045, USA
* Corresponding author.
E-mail address: john.mitchell@ucdenver.edu

Thorac Surg Clin 25 (2015) 205–215
http://dx.doi.org/10.1016/j.thorsurg.2014.12.005
1547-4127/15/$ – see front matter © 2015 Elsevier Inc. All rights reserved.

related to implementation of LDCT screening on a national level.

REVIEW OF LITERATURE EVALUATING THE COST-EFFECTIVENESS OF LOW-DOSE HELICAL COMPUTED TOMOGRAPHY SCREENING

Since the publication of the baseline screening data of the Early Lung Cancer Action Project (EL-CAP) in 1999 there has been enthusiasm for the use of LDCT in lung cancer screening. A single cohort of 1000 symptom-free volunteers, aged 60 years or older, who had at least a 10-pack-year history of smoking, was enrolled in this trial and received both a CXR and LDCT. The images were evaluated for both number and character of lung nodules and patients were referred for further work-up if radiologic criteria were met. Noncalcified nodules were either followed for growth with interval computed tomography (CT) scans or biopsied depending on size. Those found to have cancer were referred for appropriate treatment based on stage at diagnosis. One important result from this cohort of patients was that more than 80% of patients who were found to have biopsy-proven malignancy had stage I tumors at the time of diagnosis. Furthermore, LDCT scan had a cancer detection rate 4 times that of CXR (2.7% vs 0.7%).[3] The investigators theorized that, with a significant shift in the proportion of tumors that can be surgically resected and possibly cured, the long-term survival for lung cancer would improve considerably if screening with LDCT scan was adopted in high-risk individuals.

Given this potential for improved survival with LDCT screening, several studies were conducted to estimate the cost-effectiveness of adopting such a practice. These studies used a variety of statistical models to assess hypothetical cohorts of patients who are at high risk for the development of lung cancer (**Table 1**). Two studies from the same group published in 2001 simulated the effect of LDCT screening compared with no screening in a cohort of 100,000 patients aged 60 to 74 years over a 5-year period. They used the ELCAP data to inform the stage at diagnosis in the screened group and Surveillance, Epidemiology, and End Results (SEER) data to estimate stage at diagnosis in the unscreened group. The results of their first publication showed that 1-time screening with LDCT cost $5940 (1999 US dollars [USD]; $8494 in 2014 USD) per life-year saved. Accounting for a lead-time bias of 1 year, screening cost $15,274 (1999 USD; $21,842 in 2014 USD) per life-year saved assuming the EL-CAP prevalence of 2.7%.[4] The investigators performed a second analysis that expanded the

model to assess the impact of annual screening over a 5-year period. This impact increased the cost to $61,723 (1999 USD; $88,268 in 2014 USD) per life-year saved.[5] The conclusion of both articles was that LDCT screening for lung cancer seems to be cost-effective in a high-risk, elderly population. The investigators of ELCAP performed their own cost analysis shortly after the publication of their baseline results. They used a decision analysis model to estimate the costs associated with the screening CT scans and all associated follow-up procedures/treatment and then compared them with the estimated costs of lung cancer treatment in an unscreened group. They also concluded that screening with LDCT was cost-effective, with an estimated cost of $2500 per life-year gained.[6]

In contrast, 2 other simulation modeling studies published in a similar time period found that screening with LDCT was unlikely to be cost-effective.[7,8] Mahadevia and colleagues[7] used a computer-simulated model to compare 2 hypothetical cohorts of 100,000 patients. Each cohort consisted of current, quitting, and former smokers aged 60 years or older, of whom 55% were men. The screening group had a CT scan annually more than a 20-year period and a 50% stage shift in favor of earlier stage tumors was assumed. This model estimated not only that the screened cohort had 553 fewer lung cancer deaths than the unscreened cohort, but they also had significantly more invasive procedures to evaluate false-positive findings, which drove up the overall cost. The calculated incremental cost-effectiveness was $116,300 per quality-adjusted life-year (QALY) gained in current smokers and could only be reduced $42,500 per QALY if favorable estimates were used for all parameters influencing cost. Costs were even higher for quitting or former smokers. The investigators concluded that, although there was a reduction in lung cancer–specific mortality with LDCT screening, it was unlikely to be cost-effective even in elderly adult smokers. Using a similar model and hypothetical cohort, a study from Australia found that screening male current heavy smokers would only achieve acceptable cost-effectiveness ($50,000 or less) if there was a 20% reduction in lung cancer–specific mortality.[8]

Using the Lung Cancer Policy Model, a patient-level microsimulation model of lung cancer development, McMahon and colleagues[9] estimated the cost-effectiveness of CT scan screening in patient cohorts of differing ages and smoking histories. Furthermore, they evaluated the effect smoking cessation would have on cost if introduced as part of the screening program. In general, the cost of annual screening was more than $100,000 per

Table 1
Comparison of published cost analyses of screening for lung cancer with LDCT

Reference, Year Published	Marshall et al.,[4] 2001	Mahadevia et al.,[7] 2003	Manser et al.,[8] 2005	McMahon et al.,[9] 2011	Goulart et al.,[11] 2012	Pyenson et al.,[18] 2012	Villanti et al.,[10] 2013
Statistical Model	Decision analysis	Markov model	Markov model	Lung cancer policy model	Budget impact model	Actuarial analysis	Actuarial analysis
Hypothetical Cohort	100,000 patients (aged 60–74 y, 45.7% men)	100,000 patients (aged 60 y, 55% men)	10,000 patients (aged 60–64 y, 100% men)	6 cohorts, 500,000 patients in each (aged 50, 60, 70 y for men and women)	3,501,477 patients (2009 US census, assuming 6.3% eligible)	18 million insured patients (2010 US census, assuming 30% eligible)	30% of 2012 US census
Smoking History	Not reported	>20 pack y	Variable	≥20 pack y	≥30 pack y	≥30 pack y	≥30 pack y
Smoking Cessation Analysis	No	Yes	No	Yes	No	No	Yes
Frequency of Screening	One-time scan	Yearly from age 60–80 y	Yearly for 5 y	Yearly for 20 y or until age 74 y	NA	Yearly	Yearly
Basis for Stage Distribution	ELCAP	Theoretic (50% stage shift)	Weighted average of several reports	Lung cancer policy model	NLST	Theoretic	ELCAP
Helical CT Scan Cost ($)	150	300 (base) 429 (follow-up)	280	283	527	247	210
Cost-effectiveness Ratio	$5940 per life-year gained	$116,300 per QALY gained	$57,325 per life-year gained $105,090 per QALY gained	$126,000–$169,000 per QALY (20 packs/y) $110,000–$166,000 per QALY (40 packs/y)	~$240,000 per death avoided	$18,862 per life-year gained	$28,240 per QALY gained As low as $16,198 per QALY gained with smoking cessation
Author's Conclusion	CT screening is cost-effective	CT screening is not cost-effective even in heavy smokers	CT screening is unlikely to be effective unless 20% reduction in mortality	CT screening not cost-effective unless linked to smoking cessation	CT screening will add $2.0 billion in annual health care costs, but save 8000 lives per year	Cost of LDCT screening per life-year saved is favorable compared with other cancer screenings	CT screening is highly cost-effective, particularly when paired with smoking cessation

Abbreviations: NA, not available; QALY, quality-adjusted life-year.

QALY regardless of age or smoking history. However, the cost-effectiveness of screening was
significantly improved if smoking cessation
increased. CT screening has been described as a
potential teachable moment for motivating
continuing smokers to quit and, if background
quit rates doubled to 6%, cost of annual screening
for a 50-year-old patient with a minimum of 20
pack-years of smoking would decrease from
$149,000 to $73,000 per QALY.[9] Using an actuarial
model of a commercial payer system, Villanti and
colleagues[10] also showed the benefit of incorporating smoking cessation interventions with LDCT
screening. They evaluated a hypothetical cohort
of 18 million adults between ages 50 and 64 years
who had a smoking history of 30 pack-years or
greater. The cost-effectiveness of annual LDCT
screening over a 15-year period was calculated
with and without the addition of smoking cessation
interventions. Without smoking cessation interventions, the cost of screening was $28,240 per QALY
gained. With intensive smoking cessation, the cost
was reduced to $16,198 per QALY gained.

After the results of the NLST were published in
2011, Goulart and colleagues[11] estimated the
annual cost of adopting lung cancer screening in
the United States on a national level. They used
patient cohort data from the NLST and performed
an economic analysis of screening with a budget
impact model. One of the strengths of this analysis
is that the patient cohort was created by applying
the eligibility criteria from the NLST to the 2009
census. Estimates on smoking rates for patients
between the ages of 55 and 74 years were provided by the US Centers for Disease Control and
Prevention (CDC) National Health Interview Survey
(NHIS) and the Minnesota Adult Tobacco Survey.
Cost data were obtained from the Centers for
Medicare and Medicaid Service (CMS) Healthcare
Common Procedure Coding System (HCPCS).
Annual health care expenditures were calculated
as the cost of imaging studies and procedures
during diagnosis plus cancer treatment costs.
Furthermore, the cost of treating the same population without screening was subtracted from the
cost of treating those screened to obtain the
annual total expenditures attributable to
screening. Based on data from breast cancer
and colon cancer screening, the investigators estimated that only 50% to 75% of eligible patients
would reliably get screened. With this in mind,
they calculated the total annual expenditure attributable to LDCT screening as $1.303 billion and
$1.971 billion for 50% and 75% screening rates
respectively. Using the conclusion from the NLST
that 320 patients needed to be screened to prevent 1 cancer death,[1] Goulart and colleagues[11]

calculated that it would cost approximately
$240,000 per lung cancer death avoided to adopt
LDCT screening in the United States. The investigators concluded that implementation of LDCT
screening for lung cancer in the United States
would add up to $2 billion to annual national health
expenditures but also has the potential to prevent
more than 8000 lung cancer deaths per year. They
also stressed the importance of reducing false-
positive screening results (96.4% false-positive
rate in NLST) and adhering to diagnostic algorithms after a positive scan as a potential way to
reduce cost.

CALCULATION OF CURRENT ANNUAL COST OF LUNG CANCER SCREENING IN THE UNITED STATES

The budget impact assessment published by Goulart and colleagues[11] is the only analysis that is
entirely based on patients from the NLST. Given
the size and the multi-institutional design of the
trial, these data are most likely to accurately represent the cohort of patients who would be screened
if such a practice were adopted in the United
States. Current population data and lung cancer
treatment costs have been applied to the budget
impact model developed by Goulart and colleagues[11] to perform a contemporary assessment
of the annual cost of LDCT screening.

Population Eligible for Low-dose Helical Computed Tomography Screening

Data from the US 2013 census and the CDC NHIS
were used to estimate the number of patients who
would be eligible for annual LDCT screening based
on the inclusion criteria reported by the NLST. The
census data provide the number of individuals in
the United States between the ages of 55 and 74
years, whereas the NHIS estimates the prevalence
of current and former smokers within a variety of
age groups. However, the NHIS does not provide
data stratified by tobacco exposure in pack-
years. These data were estimated using an article
by Pierce and colleagues[12] published in 2011 that
used a nationwide survey to determine the percentage of moderate to heavy smokers from
1965 to 2007. Subjects were stratified by the
decade during which they were born. Greater
than 40% of subjects born between 1920 and
1930 smoked more than 10 cigarettes per day.
This decreased to between 30% and 35% for
those born between 1940 and 1960, which is the
cohort that is currently of the age allowing them
to be eligible for LDCT screening in 2014. Although
this does not give smoking data in pack-years, it is
reasonable to assume that most moderate to

heavy smokers ($\geq$10 cigarettes per day) from that time period would have accumulated 30 pack-years by 2014. Given that others[11] have estimated a heavy smoking prevalence closer to 10%, a prevalence of 20% was used for the calculations in this report. Based on previous reports of rates of screening for colon and breast cancer,[11,13] calculations assuming only 75% and 50% screening rates were performed in addition to 100%.

Health Resource Use Related to Low-dose Helical Computed Tomography Screening

To determine the annual number of patients with a positive LDCT scan, the proportion of NLST subjects with a positive scan on the second year of screening (27.9%) was multiplied by the number of those eligible. The second year of screening was used to reflect a steady state of prevalent and incident cases. This number was then multiplied by the false-positive rate (96.4%) from the trial to determine the number of patients with false-positive screening tests. The difference between the number of patients with a positive LDCT scan and those with a false-positive result was calculated as the number of patients with true-positive, screen-detected lung cancer. For those with a positive LDCT screening test, the number of confirmatory imaging studies, percutaneous biopsies, and surgical procedures were calculated using the proportions reported in the NLST. Tumor stage distribution of the 1060 confirmed lung cancer cases from the LDCT arm was applied to estimate the number of cases detected through screening. The TNM (tumor, node, metastasis) staging reported in the NLST was reclassified into localized (stage I and II), regional (stage III), and distant (stage IV) so that it could be directly compared with current SEER data that were used to estimate the distribution of cases that would occur in the same cohort without screening. This method allows a comparison between the stage distribution in screen-detected cases and the current stage distribution of nonscreened lung cancer cases in the United States.

Annual Health Care Expenditures

Health care expenditures were derived from Goulart and colleagues,[11] who used the CMS HCPCS and Diagnostic Related Group codes together to obtain the unit costs for the tests, procedures, and complications that followed a positive LDCT scan. No specific reimbursement has been set for LDCT screening, so the reimbursement rate for a conventional noncontrast chest CT was used. All expenditures consist of the product of the unit cost of the health care resource and the number

of patients who used that resource. The net treatment expenditures related to LDCT screening were calculated as the difference between the cost of treating screen-detected cases and the cost of treating those that would have been diagnosed without screening. Because screening introduces a certain percentage of overdiagnosis, or disease diagnosed by screening that would otherwise not have been detected during an individual's lifetime, all rates of lung cancer detection in the unscreened group were corrected for this factor. A recent analysis of the NLST suggested that there was an overdiagnosis rate of 18.5% in the trial,[14] so this value was used for all calculations. The cost of lung cancer treatment after diagnosis was based on a recent study of costs in Medicare enrollees.[15] The costs were broken up by year of treatment, with the initial year and last year of life being the most expensive. Years of ongoing treatment tended to be much less costly. Because this analysis is meant to only represent 1 year of cost, the cost of the last year of life was used for those with distant disease; an average of the first and last year of life was used for those with regional disease; and a weighted average of the first, ongoing, and last years of life were used for those with localized disease, assuming a median survival of 5 years.[16]

The cost per lung cancer death avoided was determined by dividing the additional costs accumulated by LDCT screening by the number of lung cancer deaths avoided by screening per year (320). The cost per life-year gained was determined by calculating the number of years a patient would live based on the stage at diagnosis. Based on the SEER data, it could be roughly estimated that a patient with localized disease would live 5 years, a patient with regional disease would live 2 years, and a patient with distant disease would only live 1 year.[16] The total number of life-years in the screened group is determined by multiplying the number of patients at each stage by the number of years they would be expected to live and then calculating the sum of those values. The same calculation can be done for the nonscreened group and then subtracted from the total number of life-years in the screened group to get the number of life-years gained by screening. The cost attributed to screening is then divided by the number of life-years gained to determine the cost per life-year gained. The cost per QALY gained was calculated using methods described previously.[17]

Results of Calculation

In the US 2013 census, there were 64,533,197 persons between the ages of 55 and 74 years. The

NHIS data suggest that the prevalence of current smokers in the age group is 17.6% and that of former smokers is 28.8%. Assuming that only 20% of smokers smoke 30 or more pack-years in a lifetime, only 3.5% (2,258,662) and 5.8% (3,742,925) of the total population would be considered current heavy smokers and former heavy smokers respectively. Therefore, 6,001,587 persons would have been eligible for screening in 2013 (**Table 2**).

Given the positive and false-positive screening rates from the NLST, approximately 1% of patients in the screened group had true-positive results from their LDCT scans. The numbers of additional tests or procedures that were performed as a result of an initial positive screening examination are outlined in **Table 3**. The most common follow-up test performed after a positive test was an additional chest CT, with the second most common being a CXR. Comparing characteristics of screen-detected cancers with those diagnosed without screening, there is shift from distant stage to localized stage in the screened group. More than half (57.1%) of screen-detected cases are in the localized stage, whereas almost two-thirds (63%) of cases in the unscreened group are in the distant stage. The proportion of regional stage cases is similar in both groups (21.2% vs 22%). The numbers of lung cancer cases diagnosed in the screened groups as well as the unscreened cohort are outlined in **Table 4**. These numbers are not equal because those in the unscreened group have been corrected for overdiagnosis.[14]

The costs attributed to the screening LDCT scans as well as follow-up imaging and procedures are shown in **Table 5** for the various screening rates. These costs range from $2.4 billion to $4.8 billion depending on the rate of LDCT screening. The costs attributable to CT scans alone are responsible for approximately 75% of this total regardless of screening rate. The expenditures attributed to treatment of lung cancer at the 3 different stages are shown in the lower half of **Table 5**. It is less costly to treat a patient with localized cancer than it is to treat either regional or distant disease. For this reason, the stage shift that accompanies each of the screened groups significantly reduces the corresponding cost of cancer treatment, as shown by the treatment cost offset by screening (see second to last row in **Table 5**). This value was calculated by taking the difference of the total treatment cost without screening and the treatment costs at each screening rate. If 100% of eligible patients underwent screening, the lung cancer treatment costs would be reduced by $1.3 billion annually. The annual total expenditures attributable to LDCT screening were calculated by subtracting the treatment cost offset by screening from the total imaging and procedural expenditures. Depending on the rate of screening, this value is between $1.7 billion and $3.4 billion (see **Table 5**). The cost per lung cancer death avoided is approximately $180,000 and the cost per life-year gained is slightly more than $28,000. When calculated for QALY, the cost per life-year gained is approximately $35,000 (**Table 6**). This value is slightly higher than that for breast and colon cancer[18] but is considerably less than the historically accepted cost of $50,000 per life-year gained used to determine the cost-effectiveness of screening examinations.[19]

AREAS FOR IMPROVEMENT

The results of the NLST suggest that widespread screening of patients who are at high risk for development of lung cancer would save many lives. However, the cost of such a program may be prohibitive in an era of rapidly escalating health care costs combined with a desire by the federal government to limit spending. Although the calculations performed in this report suggest that implementing screening for lung cancer would cost up to $3.4 billion, there are many ways that this cost could be reduced. Costs of both

Table 2
Population eligible for screening based on NLST criteria

Population Eligible for Screening	%	N (100% Screening Rate)	N (75% Screening Rate)	N (50% Screening Rate)
Aged 55–74 y in 2013 census	—	64,533,197	64,533,197	64,533,197
Prevalence of current smokers ≥30 ppy	3.5	2,258,662	1,693,997	1,129,331
Prevalence of former smokers ≥30 ppy	5.8	3,742,925	2,807,194	1,871,463
Population screened	9.3	6,001,587	4,501,191	3,000,794

Abbreviation: ppy, packs per year.

Data from Aberle DR, Adams AM, Berg CD, et al. Reduced lung-cancer mortality with low-dose computed tomographic screening. N Engl J Med 2011;365(5):395–409.

Table 3
Screening test performance and health resource use

	%	N (100% Screening Rate)	N (75% Screening Rate)	N (50% Screening Rate)
Screening Test Performance				
Positive screening rate	27.9	1,674,443	1,255,832	837,222
False-positive rate	26.9	1,614,427	1,210,820	807,214
True-positive rate	1.0	60,015	45,013	30,009
Health Resource Use (Imaging/Procedures)				
Positive LDCT	100	1,674,443	1,255,832	837,222
Follow-up CXR	14.4	241,120	180,840	120,560
Follow-up chest CT	49.8	833,873	625,404	416,937
Follow-up PET/CT	8.3	138,979	104,234	69,489
Percutaneous biopsy	1.8	30,140	22,605	15,070
Bronchoscopy without biopsy	1.8	30,140	22,605	15,070
Bronchoscopy with biopsy	2.2	36,838	25,117	18,419
Mediastinoscopy	0.7	11,721	8791	5861
Thoracoscopy	1.3	21,768	16,326	10,884
Thoracotomy	2.9	48,559	36,419	24,279
Major complications	0.5	8372	6279	4186
Intermediate Complications	0.8	13,396	10,047	6698

Adapted from Aberle DR, Adams AM, Berg CD, et al. Reduced lung-cancer mortality with low-dose computed tomographic screening. N Engl J Med 2011;365(5):395–409.

Table 4
Number of lung cancer cases diagnosed

Lung Cancer Cases: Screening Adopted	Rate (%)	N (100% Screening)	N (75% Screening)	N (50% Screening)
Screening-detected Cases				
Localized	57.1	34,269	25,702	17,135
Regional	21.2	12,723	9543	6362
Distant	21.7	13,023	9768	6512
Total cases	100.0	60,015	45,013	30,009
Cases in Patients Who Missed Screening[a]				
Localized	15.0	0	1834	3669
Regional	22.0	0	2690	5381
Distant	63.0	0	7704	15,408
Total cases	100.0	0	12,228	24,458
Lung Cancer Cases: Screening Not Adopted	**Rate (%)**	**N (100% Screening)**	**N (75% Screening)**	**N (50% Screening)**
Localized	15.0	—	7337	—
Regional	22.0	—	10,761	—
Distant	63.0	—	30,815	—
Total Cases	100.0	—	48,913	—

[a] Stage distribution based on SEER data,[16] corrected for 18.5% overdiagnosis.[14]
Data from National Cancer Institute. Surveillance epidemiology and end results. National Institute of Health. 2013. Available at: http://seer.cancer.gov/. Accessed August 14, 2014; and Patz EF Jr, Pinsky P, Gatsonis C, et al. Overdiagnosis in low-dose computed tomography screening for lung cancer. JAMA Intern Med 2014;174:269–74.

Table 5
Annual Health Care Expenditures Attributable to Low-Dose CT Screening

Health Care Resource	Unit Cost (2011 US$)	Expenditures w/ 100% Screening (US$ Millions)	Expenditures w/ 75% Screening (US$ Millions)	Expenditures w/ 50% Screening (US$ Millions)	Expenditures with no Screening (US$ Millions)
LDCT scan	527	3,162.8	2,372.1	1,581.4	N/A
F/up CXR	92	22.2	16.6	11.1	N/A
F/up Chest CT	527	439.5	329.6	219.7	N/A
F/up PET/CT	1,491	207.2	155.4	103.6	N/A
Percutaneous biopsy	979	29.5	22.1	14.8	N/A
Bronchoscopy w/out biopsy	1,226	37.0	27.7	18.5	N/A
Bronchoscopy w/biopsy	1,270	46.8	31.9	23.4	N/A
Mediastinoscopy	3,814	44.7	33.5	22.4	N/A
Thoracoscopy	3,795	82.6	62.0	41.3	N/A
Thoracotomy	11,285	548.0	411.0	274.0	N/A
Major complications	10,096	84.5	63.4	42.3	N/A
Intermediate complications	6,072	81.3	61.0	40.7	N/A
Total imaging and procedure expenditures		4,786.1	3,586.3	2,393.2	N/A

Treatment expenditures in screen-detected cases					
Localized stage	35,648.6	1,221.6	916.2	610.8	N/A
Regional stage	107,096.5	1,362.6	1,022.0	681.3	N/A
Distant stage	141,300.2	1,840.2	1,380.2	920.1	N/A
Treatment expenditures for those who missed screening					
Localized stage	35,648.6	0	65.4	130.8	N/A
Regional stage	107,096.5	0	288.1	576.3	N/A
Distant stage	141,300.2	0	1,088.6	2,177.2	N/A
Total screening treatment expenditures		**4,424.4**	**4,688.5**	**5,096.5**	**N/A**
Treatment if screening not adopted					
Localized stage	35,648.6			261.6	
Regional stage	107,096.5			1152.5	
Distant stage	141,300.2			4354.2	
Total treatment cost if no screening				**5768.3**	
Treatment cost offset by screening		1,343.9	1,079.8	671.8	N/A
Annual total Expenditures attributable to LDCT screening		**3,442.2**	**2,506.5**	**1,721.4**	**N/A**

Table 6
Cost-effectiveness calculations

	100% Screening Rate	75% Screening Rate	50% Screening Rate
Cost per Lung Cancer Death Avoided (US$)	183,535	178,196	183,577
Life-years Saved by Screening	120,792	90,596	60,408
Cost per Life-year Saved (US$)	28,497	27,667	28,496
Cost per QALY Saved (US$)	35,577	34,540	35,576

screening and diagnostic CT scans of the chest make up most of the cost of screening. In this report, a cost of $527 for a CT scan of the chest was used. This value was derived from a previous publication[11] that used the values on the CMS Web site to determine cost. Other publications have reported the cost of noncontrast CT of the chest as being as low as $150. If this value was applied to the calculations in this report, the total cost attributable to screening would be less than $900 million, assuming that 100% of eligible patients were screened. If a more realistic value of $250 is used, the cost attributable to screening would only come up to approximately $1.5 billion annually, which would mean that the cost per lung cancer death avoided would come down to $83,000 and the cost per life-year gained would be $13,000, putting screening with LDCT at a level of cost-effectiveness that is on par with screening for breast and colon cancer.[18]

The false-positive rate from the screening scans in the NLST led to a large number of unnecessary procedures and imaging studies. The NLST began accrual in 2002 at a time when CT scan technology was far behind where it is currently. As the technology has improved, the use of volumetric assessment of nodules to better quantify interval growth helps restrict invasive diagnostic work-up to more aggressive screen-detected tumors.[20,21] In addition, the follow-up of suspicious nodules in the NLST was left to community standards rather than being optimized before proceeding with the trial, which may have led to more invasive and less effective follow-up and ultimately increased cost. If widespread implementation of LDCT scanning for lung cancer screening is to occur, using

contemporary CT scan technology and establishing a best practice for the screening follow-up could considerably reduce cost.

The use of annual LDCT screening as a teachable moment for physicians to stress the negative effects of smoking could reduce costs considerably if rates of smoking cessation increase.[9,10] A study from the ELCAP showed that 23% of active smokers reported quitting after a baseline CT scan; a rate that is more than 4 times greater than the background quit rate in the general population.[22] By preventing patients from developing cancer with smoking cessation, the cost of diagnostic imaging and procedures is reduced. Furthermore, estimating coronary artery calcium scores and grading emphysema can promote personalized medicine and further maximize teachable moments.

PAYMENT FOR LUNG CANCER SCREENING

A provision of the Patient Protection and Affordable Care Act requires that most insurers provide coverage, without cost sharing (deductible or copayment), for preventative care services that receive an A or B recommendation from the USPSTF. LDCT scanning for lung cancer screening has received a B-rated recommendation and therefore should be covered under this mandate. As of October, 2014, a decision from CMS as to whether Medicare will cover this service has not yet been made. Earlier this same year, the Medicare Evidence and Coverage Advisory Committee voted against recommending national Medicare coverage for annual screening for lung cancer with LDCT. One argument against Medicare coverage is that almost 75% of participants in the NLST were less than 65 years of age. Some committee members thought that the results may not translate to the Medicare population; however, a recent publication comparing the cohort less than 65 years old with the cohort 65 years and older from the NLST suggests otherwise.[23] The investigators found that the lung cancer prevalence was higher in the older cohort and that the number needed to screen to prevent 1 lung cancer death was lower than in the younger cohort (245 vs 364). Despite this, the cost to Medicare to cover LDCT screening has been estimated at more than $9 billion over the first 5 years,[24] and, with the current efforts to prevent spending by the federal government, CMS may find that it is too costly to cover at this time.

SUMMARY

Based on the results of the NLST, the largest and most extensive single-organ cancer screening trial in history, we are certain that some lung cancer deaths can be prevented with LDCT screening. Given the degree to which this occurred in the trial, widespread use of LDCT screening is likely to occur. The cost of implementing such a screening program is likely to be considerable, but remains unknown. The estimates from this report based on the NLST data suggest that the cost would be between $2 billion and $4 billion, depending on screening rates. As CT scanning technology improves and best-practice guidelines for follow-up are established, this cost is likely to come down, making LDCT a cost-effective method of preventing lung cancer death in the United States.

REFERENCES

1. National Lung Screening Trial Research Team, Aberle DR, Adams AM, et al. Reduced lung-cancer mortality with low-dose computed tomographic screening. N England J Med 2011;365:395–409.

2. Moyer VA, US Preventive Services Task Force. Screening for lung cancer: U.S. Preventive Services Task Force recommendation statement. Ann Intern Med 2014;160:330–8.

3. Henschke CI, McCauley DI, Yankelevitz DF, et al. Early lung cancer action project: overall design and findings from baseline screening. Lancet 1999;354:99–105.

4. Marshall D, Simpson KN, Earle CC, et al. Potential cost-effectiveness of one-time screening for lung cancer (LC) in a high risk cohort. Lung Cancer 2001;32:227–36.

5. Marshall D, Simpson KN, Earle CC, et al. Economic decision analysis model of screening for lung cancer. Eur J Cancer 2001;37:1759–67.

6. Wisnivesky JP, Mushlin AI, Sicherman N, et al. The cost-effectiveness of low-dose CT screening for lung cancer: preliminary results of baseline screening. Chest 2003;124:614–21.

7. Mahadevia PJ, Fleisher LA, Frick KD, et al. Lung cancer screening with helical computed tomography in older adult smokers: a decision and cost-effectiveness analysis. JAMA 2003;289:313–22.

8. Manser R, Dalton A, Carter R, et al. Cost-effectiveness analysis of screening for lung cancer with low dose spiral CT (computed tomography) in the Australian setting. Lung Cancer 2005;48:171–85.

9. McMahon PM, Kong CY, Bouzan C, et al. Cost-effectiveness of computed tomography screening for lung cancer in the United States. J Thorac Oncol 2011;6:1841–8.

10. Villanti AC, Jiang Y, Abrams DB, et al. A cost-utility analysis of lung cancer screening and the additional

11. Goulart BH, Bensink ME, Mummy DG, et al. Lung cancer screening with low-dose computed tomography: costs, national expenditures, and cost-effectiveness. J Natl Compr Canc Netw 2012;10:267–75.

12. Pierce JP, Messer K, White MM, et al. Prevalence of heavy smoking in California and the United States, 1965-2007. JAMA 2011;305:1106–12.

13. Breen N, Gentleman JF, Schiller JS. Update on mammography trends: comparisons of rates in 2000, 2005, and 2008. Cancer 2011;117:2209–18.

14. Patz EF Jr, Pinsky P, Gatsonis C, et al. Overdiagnosis in low-dose computed tomography screening for lung cancer. JAMA Intern Med 2014;174:269–74.

15. Mariotto AB, Yabroff KR, Shao Y, et al. Projections of the cost of cancer care in the United States: 2010-2020. J Natl Cancer Inst 2011;103:117–28.

16. National Cancer Institute. Surveillance epidemiology and end results. Bethesda (MD): National Institute of Health; 2013. Available at: http://seer.cancer.gov/. Accessed August 14, 2014.

17. Hanmer J, Lawrence WF, Anderson JP, et al. Report of nationally representative values for the noninstitutionalized US adult population for 7 health-related quality-of-life scores. Med Decis Making 2006;26:391–400.

18. Pyenson BS, Sander MS, Jiang Y, et al. An actuarial analysis shows that offering lung cancer screening as an insurance benefit would save lives at relatively low cost. Health Aff 2012;31:770–9.

19. Braithwaite RS, Meltzer DO, King JT Jr, et al. What does the value of modern medicine say about the $50,000 per quality-adjusted life-year decision rule? Med Care 2008;46:349–56.

20. Mulshine JL, Jablons DM. Volume CT for diagnosis of nodules found in lung-cancer screening. N Engl J Med 2009;361:2281–2.

21. van Klaveren RJ, Oudkerk M, Prokop M, et al. Management of lung nodules detected by volume CT scanning. N Engl J Med 2009;361:2221–9.

22. Ostroff JS, Buckshee N, Mancuso CA, et al. Smoking cessation following CT screening for early detection of lung cancer. Prev Med 2001;33:613–21.

23. Pinsky PF, Gierada DS, Hocking W, et al. National lung screening trial findings by age: Medicare-eligible versus under-65 population. Ann Intern Med 2014;161(9):627–33.

24. Roth JA, Sullivan SD, Ravelo A, et al. Low-dose computed tomography lung cancer screening in the Medicare program: projected clinical, resource, and budget impact. J Clin Oncol 2014;32(15 suppl):6501.

Refining Strategies to Identify Populations to Be Screened for Lung Cancer

Ugo Pastorino, MD[a],*, Mario Silva, MD[a,b]

KEYWORDS

- Lung cancer • Screening • Biological sampling • Imaging

KEY POINTS

- The selection of populations to be screened for lung cancer must be further optimized before translation to large population.
- A 3-step refinement should be integrated into forthcoming lung cancer trials, namely, calculation of risk based on (1) demographics, (2) biological factors, and (3) radiologic inputs.
- Biological sampling should be implemented up-front to reduce the use of low-dose computed tomography scanning in patients with lower risk of aggressive disease and, notably, to detect aggressive disease that is overlooked by current screening strategies.

In the past 20 years, lung cancer screening trials have been performed with a high detection rate, notably for early-stage disease.[1] Imaging has always played a pivotal role in such screening programs, under the axiom of correlation between pulmonary nodule and lung cancer.[2] The introduction of low-dose computed tomography (LDCT) allowed for sensitive detection of extremely small pulmonary nodules.[3–23] Therefore, LDCT has been advocated as a sensitive tool for diagnosing early lung cancer and, therefore, improvement of survival. The National Lung Screening Trial (NLST) reported a 20% reduction of deaths from lung cancer in smokers, compared with the chest radiography control group.[24] This striking result is in contrast with data reported by smaller European trials, which have not shown a clear-cut advantage of LDCT screening over observational strategies.[25–27]

Since the beginning of computed tomography–based lung cancer screening trials, the detection of a solid nodule measuring 5 mm or greater has

been deemed a predictive factor of lung cancer and, therefore, worthy of further investigation. This approach led to a significant increase of LDCT and invasive procedures, and, therefore, radiation exposure, risks, and health care costs. An open debate exists about the overwhelming predominance of false-positive LDCT findings[28,29] and their implications in large-population lung cancer screening (ie, anxiety, radiation exposure, diagnostic workups and the related complications).[29] In the past 2 years, data have been published about possible strategies to reduce the workup resulting from LDCT false-positive findings, while keeping the high sensitivity of LDCT.

The International Early Lung Cancer Action Project (I-ELCAP) and NLST tested the effects of using a progressively higher nodule size threshold and demonstrated a potential decrease of 34% to 75% in LDCT examinations with minimal delay in diagnosis and treatment of lung cancer.[30,31] The new guidelines issued by the American College

The authors have nothing to disclose.

[a] Division of Thoracic Surgery, Istituto Nazionale Tumori, Via Venezian 1, Milan 20133, Italy; [b] Section of Radiology, Department of Surgical Sciences, University of Parma, Via Gramsci 14, Parma 43126, Italy
* Corresponding author.
E-mail address: ugo.pastorino@istitutotumori.mi.it

Thorac Surg Clin 25 (2015) 217–221
http://dx.doi.org/10.1016/j.thorsurg.2014.11.005
1547-4127/15/$ – see front matter © 2015 Elsevier Inc. All rights reserved.

of Radiology reflect the awareness that a larger size threshold (ie, 6 mm) may be appropriate for nodule management within lung cancer screening programs.[32] Further optimization of screening programs could be gained through volumetric measurement of nodules. A recent report from the NELSON (Nederlands Leuvens Screening Onderzoek) trial showed that lung nodules smaller than 100 mm^3 were not predictive of lung cancer in the following 2 years (ie, 2-year lung cancer risk of 0.6% vs 0.4% in subjects without nodules). Moreover, they calculated a 2-year lung cancer risk of 2.4% for subjects with nodules measuring 100 to 300 mm^3 (intermediate risk) and 16.9% for those with nodules greater than 300 mm^3 (high risk).[33] Accordingly, they proposed volume-doubling time (VDT) assessment of nodules measuring 100 to 300 mm^3 or immediate diagnostic investigation of nodules greater than 300 mm^3. In particular, the 2-year risk of lung cancer was shown to be 4% for VDTs of 400 to 600 days and 9.9% for VDTs of 400 days or less.[33] These results are a huge step toward higher positive predictive values of lung cancer screening.

Furthermore, not only positive predictive value (malignant vs benign) but also overdiagnosis (indolent vs aggressive tumor) was brought to the attention of lung cancer screening panelists.[34,35] In the era of LDCT lung cancer screening trials, a significant increase in detection of early-stage indolent tumors has been reported without an apportioned decrease in detection of aggressive tumors.[36] This shift to slow-growing cancers is the most likely explanation for the almost equal mortality seen in the LDCT and chest radiography arms, despite a significant increase in prevalence of resectable early-stage cancers in the former.[34] Therefore, further characterization should be sought to increase lung cancer screening accuracy.

Biomarkers have been proposed for the early detection of lung cancer.[37,38] In particular, microRNA (miRNA) has been shown to have abnormal expression in most types of cancer.[39] Specific patterns of miRNAs expression have been demonstrated in the primary tumor and the blood, thus suggesting that circulating miRNAs provide disease fingerprints.[40,41] The implementation of these markers in LDCT screening programs has been proposed to inform the optimization of protocols according to risk profiles based on miRNA patterns.[28,42] Specific serologic miRNA patterns have been tested in the selection of high-risk subjects within lung cancer screening trials.[43,44] The authors' group showed a significant association between a miRNA signature classifier (MSC) and lung cancer in retrospective analyses of circulating miRNAs, which were prospectively collected

within the randomized Multicenter Italian Lung Detection (MILD) trial.[45] The high sensitivity and negative predictive value of MSC fostered a newly designed protocol for a second trial, the so-called bioMILD trial. (MSCs used in bioMILD consist of reciprocal quantification of 24 circulating miRNAs). In bioMILD, the LDCT protocol was designed to reduce the number of scans while providing dedicated surveillance to subjects with a higher risk of lung cancer. In particular, participants of bioMILD undergo blood sampling and LDC at baseline and each designated round. The evaluation of MSC provides comprehensive risk stratification and, therefore, selection of a dedicated LDCT follow-up strategy, either in 1 or 3 years. The number of LDCT scans is by default reduced to one-third in subjects with low risk, resulting in a substantial reduction in radiographic exposure for subjects who would not benefit from yearly LDCT. On the other hand, subjects at higher risk are maintained on yearly LDCT follow-up.

Furthermore, this trial integrates a risk stratification system, and therefore follow-up strategy, based on nodule features. The implementation of serologic miRNA sampling allowed for an increasing volumetric threshold for nodules, thus providing even lower recall rate based on nodule size. This strategy derives from the simulation performed on the MILD population, wherein the assessment of lung cancer risk using an MSC would have allowed for a 5-fold reduction of false-positive findings for nodules measuring 5 mm or greater (from 19.4% to 3.7%). Furthermore, a correlation was observed between interval cancers and MSC risk category. In the MILD trial, 8 of 9 (89%) subjects with interval cancer were categorized as MSC intermediate-high risk.[45] Because interval cancer remains an issue in lung cancer screening, the results of the bioMILD trial are anticipated to determine whether MSC could increase the early detection of cancers that are overlooked by current screening strategies.

MSC and LDCT together were retrospectively tested in MILD and showed a 98% cumulative sensitivity (57 of 58 cancers), whereas the sensitivity of each test alone was 87% and 84%, respectively. Furthermore, MSC risk category predicted a shorter 3-year survival; therefore, subjects with a confirmed high risk by MSC are selected for additional workup to exclude extrapulmonary causes of mortality. Another lung cancer screening program in Milan is using the miRNA test, namely the Cosmos-II trial. In this study, the 1-year risk of lung cancer is rated according to demographic risk models, with the selection of 2 main populations. In particular, participants with

1-year cancer risk less than 0.6% are enrolled in a biennial LDCT screening arm, whereas subjects with a risk of 0.6% or greater are tested with annual LDCT and sampling of circulating miRNA.[46] The main difference between the bioMILD and Cosmos-II strategies is the criteria for selecting high-risk patients: bioMILD uses circulating miRNA samples as an up-front test in all recruited participants, whereas Cosmos-II tests miRNA in just a portion of participants. The advantage of using miRNA sampling as an up-front test is the comprehensive classification of both the risk of lung cancer and the likelihood of having a diagnosis of lung cancer in the next 3 years. Furthermore, MSC allows for the selection of subjects at high risk of aggressive lung cancer.[45] Therefore, specific characterization of risks is provided by miRNA compared with demographic risk models.

Still, demographic risk models are needed for the first-level selection of populations appropriate for lung cancer screening in order to optimize costs. A difference is seen in cancer prevalence among trials that include nonsmokers and those dedicated to current and recently former smokers, thus showing the substantial increase in lung cancer detection in subjects with demographic risk factors.[47] Screening panelists have proposed several demographic models of lung cancer risk with the purpose of reducing unnecessary LDCT and increasing efficacy.[48–52] In 2003, Bach and colleagues[48] advocated the evaluation of specific lung cancer risk among smokers. In 2013, Tammemagi and colleagues[52] proposed selection criteria for lung cancer screening according to lung cancer risk models derived from the analyses of 80,375 PLCO participants. The United Kingdom Lung Cancer Screening trial (UKLS) has an original strategy designed to screen subjects with a lung cancer risk of 5% or greater in 5 years according to the Liverpool Lung Project risk model.[51,53] The UKLS uses the Wald Single Screen Design, which is optimized for cost and long-term compliance, but also provides complete data for planning subsequent screens.[53] The results of this alternative study are anticipated.

In conclusion, the selection of populations to be screened for lung cancer must be further optimized before translation to large population. A 3-step refinement should be integrated into forthcoming lung cancer trials, namely, calculation of risk based on (1) demographics, (2) biological factors, and (3) radiologic inputs. Biological sampling should be implemented up-front to reduce the use of LDCT scanning in patients with lower risk of aggressive disease and, notably, to detect aggressive disease that is overlooked by current screening strategies.

REFERENCES

1. Bach PB, Jett JR, Pastorino U, et al. Computed tomography screening and lung cancer outcomes. JAMA 2007;297(9):953–61.
2. Melamed MR, Flehinger BJ. Screening for lung cancer. Chest 1984;86(1):2–3.
3. Henschke CI, McCauley DI, Yankelevitz DF, et al. Early lung cancer action project: overall design and findings from baseline screening. Lancet 1999;354(9173):99–105.
4. Sone S, Li F, Yang ZG, et al. Results of three-year mass screening programme for lung cancer using mobile low-dose spiral computed tomography scanner. Br J Cancer 2001;84(1):25–32.
5. Nawa T, Nakagawa T, Kusano S, et al. Lung cancer screening using low-dose spiral CT: results of baseline and 1-year follow-up studies. Chest 2002; 122(1):15–20.
6. Sobue T, Moriyama N, Kaneko M, et al. Screening for lung cancer with low-dose helical computed tomography: anti-lung cancer association project. J Clin Oncol 2002;20(4):911–20.
7. Pastorino U, Bellomi M, Landoni C, et al. Early lung-cancer detection with spiral CT and positron emission tomography in heavy smokers: 2-year results. Lancet 2003;362(9384):593–7.
8. Swensen SJ, Jett JR, Hartman TE, et al. Lung cancer screening with CT: Mayo Clinic experience. Radiology 2003;226(3):756–61.
9. Diederich S, Thomas M, Semik M, et al. Screening for early lung cancer with low-dose spiral computed tomography: results of annual follow-up examinations in asymptomatic smokers. Eur Radiol 2004; 14(4):691–702.
10. Bastarrika G, Garcia-Velloso MJ, Lozano MD, et al. Early lung cancer detection using spiral computed tomography and positron emission tomography. Am J Respir Crit Care Med 2005;171(12):1378–83.
11. Chong S, Lee KS, Chung MJ, et al. Lung cancer screening with low-dose helical CT in Korea: experiences at the Samsung Medical Center. J Korean Med Sci 2005;20(3):402–8.
12. Gohagan JK, Marcus PM, Fagerstrom RM, et al. Final results of the Lung Screening Study, a randomized feasibility study of spiral CT versus chest X-ray screening for lung cancer. Lung Cancer 2005;47(1): 9–15.
13. Novello S, Fava C, Borasio P, et al. Three-year findings of an early lung cancer detection feasibility study with low-dose spiral computed tomography in heavy smokers. Ann Oncol 2005;16(10):1662–6.
14. MacRedmond R, McVey G, Lee M, et al. Screening for lung cancer using low dose CT scanning: results of 2 year follow up. Thorax 2006;61(1):54–6.
15. Callol L, Roig F, Cuevas A, et al. Low-dose CT: a useful and accessible tool for the early diagnosis

of lung cancer in selected populations. Lung Cancer 2007;56(2):217–21.

16. Infante M, Lutman FR, Cavuto S, et al. Lung cancer screening with spiral CT: baseline results of the randomized DANTE trial. Lung Cancer 2008;59(3): 355–63.

17. van den Bergh KA, Essink-Bot ML, Bunge EM, et al. Impact of computed tomography screening for lung cancer on participants in a randomized controlled trial (NELSON trial). Cancer 2008;113(2):396–404.

18. Veronesi G, Bellomi M, Mulshine JL, et al. Lung cancer screening with low-dose computed tomography: a non-invasive diagnostic protocol for baseline lung nodules. Lung Cancer 2008;61(3):340–9.

19. Wilson DO, Weissfeld JL, Fuhrman CR, et al. The Pittsburgh Lung Screening Study (PLuSS): outcomes within 3 years of a first computed tomography scan. Am J Respir Crit Care Med 2008;178(9): 956–61.

20. Lopes Pegna A, Picozzi G, Mascalchi M, et al. Design, recruitment and baseline results of the ITA-LUNG trial for lung cancer screening with low-dose CT. Lung Cancer 2009;64(1):34–40.

21. Pedersen JH, Ashraf H, Dirksen A, et al. The Danish randomized lung cancer CT screening trial–overall design and results of the prevalence round. J Thorac Oncol 2009;4(5):608–14.

22. Menezes RJ, Roberts HC, Paul NS, et al. Lung cancer screening using low-dose computed tomography in at-risk individuals: the Toronto experience. Lung Cancer 2010;67(2):177–83.

23. Becker N, Motsch E, Gross ML, et al. Randomized study on early detection of lung cancer with MSCT in Germany: study design and results of the first screening round. J Cancer Res Clin Oncol 2012; 138(9):1475–86.

24. National Lung Screening Trial Research Team, Aberle DR, Adams AM, et al. Reduced lung-cancer mortality with low-dose computed tomographic screening. N Engl J Med 2011;365(5):395–409.

25. Infante M, Cavuto S, Lutman FR, et al. A randomized study of lung cancer screening with spiral computed tomography: three-year results from the DANTE trial. Am J Respir Crit Care Med 2009;180(5):445–53.

26. Saghir Z, Dirksen A, Ashraf H, et al. CT screening for lung cancer brings forward early disease. The randomised Danish lung cancer screening trial: status after five annual screening rounds with low-dose CT. Thorax 2012;67(4):296–301.

27. Pastorino U, Rossi M, Rosato V, et al. Annual or biennial CT screening versus observation in heavy smokers: 5-year results of the MILD trial. Eur J Cancer Prev 2012;21(3):308–15.

28. Goulart BH, Bensink ME, Mummy DG, et al. Lung cancer screening with low-dose computed tomography: costs, national expenditures, and cost-effectiveness. J Natl Compr Canc Netw 2012;10(2):267–75.

29. Woolf SH, Harris RP, Campos-Outcalt D. Low-dose computed tomography screening for lung cancer: how strong is the evidence? JAMA Intern Med 2014;174(12):2019–22.

30. Henschke CI, Yip R, Yankelevitz DF, et al, International Early Lung Cancer Action Program Investigators. Definition of a positive test result in computed tomography screening for lung cancer: a cohort study. Ann Intern Med 2013;158(4):246–52.

31. Yip R, Henschke CI, Yankelevitz DF, et al. CT screening for lung cancer: alternative definitions of positive test result based on the National Lung Screening Trial and International Early Lung Cancer Action Program databases. Radiology 2014;273(2): 591–6.

32. American College of Radiology. Lung-RADS Version 1.0 Assessment Categories Release date: April 28, 2014. Available at: http://www.acr.org/~/media/ACR/Documents/PDF/QualitySafety/Resources/LungRADS/AssessmentCategories. Access May 29, 2014.

33. Horeweg N, van Rosmalen J, Heuvelmans MA, et al. Lung cancer probability in patients with CT-detected pulmonary nodules: a prespecified analysis of data from the NELSON trial of low-dose CT screening. Lancet Oncol 2014;15(12):1332–41.

34. Marcus PM, Bergstralh EJ, Zweig MH, et al. Extended lung cancer incidence follow-up in the Mayo Lung Project and overdiagnosis. J Natl Cancer Inst 2006;98(11):748–56.

35. Patz EF Jr, Pinsky P, Gatsonis C, et al. Overdiagnosis in low-dose computed tomography screening for lung cancer. JAMA Intern Med 2014;174(2):269–74.

36. Vazquez M, Carter D, Brambilla E, et al. Solitary and multiple resected adenocarcinomas after CT screening for lung cancer: histopathologic features and their prognostic implications. Lung Cancer 2009;64(2):148–54.

37. Tockman MS. Clinical detection of lung cancer progression markers. J Cell Biochem Suppl 1996;25: 177–84.

38. Lam S, Boyle P, Healey GF, et al. Early CDT-Lung: an immunobiomarker test as an aid to early detection of lung cancer. Cancer Prev Res (Phila) 2011;4(7): 1126–34.

39. Iorio MV, Croce CM. MicroRNA dysregulation in cancer: diagnostics, monitoring and therapeutics. A comprehensive review. EMBO Mol Med 2012;4(3): 143–59.

40. Chen X, Ba Y, Ma L, et al. Characterization of microRNAs in serum: a novel class of biomarkers for diagnosis of cancer and other diseases. Cell Res 2008; 18(10):997–1006.

41. Molina-Pinelo S, Pastor MD, Suarez R, et al. MicroRNA clusters: dysregulation in lung adenocarcinoma and COPD. Eur Respir J 2014;43(6):1740–9.

42. Peres J. Lung cancer screening gets risk-specific. J Natl Cancer Inst 2013;105(1):1–2.

43. Bianchi F, Nicassio F, Marzi M, et al. A serum circulating miRNA diagnostic test to identify asymptomatic high-risk individuals with early stage lung cancer. EMBO Mol Med 2011;3(8):495–503.

44. Boeri M, Verri C, Conte D, et al. MicroRNA signatures in tissues and plasma predict development and prognosis of computed tomography detected lung cancer. Proc Natl Acad Sci U S A 2011;108(9):3713–8.

45. Sozzi G, Boeri M, Rossi M, et al. Clinical utility of a plasma-based miRNA signature classifier within computed tomography lung cancer screening: a correlative MILD trial study. J Clin Oncol 2014; 32(8):768–73.

46. Filippo L, Principe R, Cesario A, et al. Smoking cessation intervention within the framework of a lung cancer screening program: preliminary results and clinical perspectives from the "Cosmos-II" trial. Lung 2014. [Epub ahead of print].

47. Pastorino U. Current status of lung cancer screening. Thorac Surg Clin 2013;23(2):129–40.

48. Bach PB, Kattan MW, Thornquist MD, et al. Variations in lung cancer risk among smokers. J Natl Cancer Inst 2003;95(6):470–8.

49. Bach PB, Elkin EB, Pastorino U, et al. Benchmarking lung cancer mortality rates in current and former smokers. Chest 2004;126(6):1742–9.

50. Spitz MR, Hong WK, Amos CI, et al. A risk model for prediction of lung cancer. J Natl Cancer Inst 2007; 99(9):715–26.

51. Cassidy A, Myles JP, van Tongeren M, et al. The LLP risk model: an individual risk prediction model for lung cancer. Br J Cancer 2008;98(2):270–6.

52. Tammemagi MC, Katki HA, Hocking WG, et al. Selection criteria for lung-cancer screening. N Engl J Med 2013;368(8):728–36.

53. Baldwin DR, Duffy SW, Wald NJ, et al. UK Lung Screen (UKLS) nodule management protocol: modelling of a single screen randomised controlled trial of low-dose CT screening for lung cancer. Thorax 2011;66(4):308–13.

Long-term Oncologic and Financial Implications of Lung Cancer Screening

Jesper Holst Pedersen, MD, DMSc[a],*, Jens Benn Sørensen, MD, DMSc, MPA[b]

KEYWORDS

- Lung cancer screening • Cost effectiveness • Oncologic implications
- Computed tomography screening future implementation

KEY POINTS

- Likely scenarios for implementation of computed tomography screening for lung cancer with focus on the screened populations and the screening method, the lung cancer detection rates, and the number of lives saved.
- Oncologic implications of computed tomography screening with focus on consequences of changes in disease stage, changes in pathology, and long-term scenarios and future research areas.
- Financial Implications of computed tomography screening with focus on costs of computed tomography screening, cost effectiveness, and long-term scenarios, including ways to increase cost effectiveness.

INTRODUCTION

Low-dose computed tomography (LDCT) screening for lung cancer has not been implemented on a national scale anywhere in the world. In the United States, the recent recommendation by the US Preventive Services Task Force (USPSTF) to implement annual lung cancer screening[1] makes it probable that in the United States, national lung cancer screening in high-risk individuals will be a reality within a few years. Knowledge of effects and consequences of lung cancer screening is currently derived from randomized trials and selected cohort studies, and therefore predictions of possible general consequences must be interpreted with caution. Nevertheless, implementation of CT screening is expected to have substantial implications for lung cancer health care and treatment. Here the authors discuss the possible scenarios for CT lung cancer screening and give some suggestions for the long-term oncologic and financial implications of its implementation.

BACKGROUND AND LIKELY SCENARIOS
The Screened Populations

The National Lung Screening Trial (NLST) randomly assigned 53,454 current or former heavy smokers to either chest radiography (CXR) or LDCT for 3 annual screenings. The NLST study documented a statistically significant reduction in overall mortality by LDCT (relative risk [RR], 0.93; 95% confidence limits (cl), 0.86–0.99) and is the only trial showing statistically significant effect on lung cancer mortality (RR, 0.80; 95% cl, 0.73–0.93).[2] The NLST enrolled participants 55 to 74 years of age at the time of randomization who had a smoking history of at least 30 pack-years

Disclosures: The authors have nothing to disclose.
[a] Department of Cardiothoracic Surgery, Rigshospitalet, University of Copenhagen, Blegdamsvej 9, Copenhagen 2100, Denmark; [b] Department of Oncology, Finsen Centre, Rigshospitalet, University of Copenhagen, Blegdamsvej 9, Copenhagen 2100, Denmark
* Corresponding author.
E-mail address: jesper.holst.pedersen@rh.regionh.dk

Thorac Surg Clin 25 (2015) 223–229
http://dx.doi.org/10.1016/j.thorsurg.2014.11.006

and were current smokers or had quit within the last 15 years.[2] The USPSTF recommends that the NLST criteria are followed, but the age limit should be extended to 80 years, and that screening should be discontinued once the individual has not smoked for 15 years.[1] The American Association for Thoracic Surgery has recommended similar selection criteria but additionally recommends screening in persons with a 20 pack-year smoking history and other conditions that produce a cumulative risk of lung cancer for at least 5% over the next 5 years in addition to lung cancer survivors 55 to 79 years of age.[3] The National Comprehensive Cancer Network recommends screening in persons ages 55 to 74 years who have at least a 30 pack-year smoking history and, if a former smoker, 15 years or less since quitting or persons ages 50 years or older who have at least a 20 pack-year smoking history and 1 additional risk factor. It does not recommend lung cancer screening in persons who are at moderate risk (age >50 years and >20 pack-year smoking history or secondhand smoke exposure but no additional lung cancer risk factors) or low risk (younger than 50 years or smoking history of <20 pack-years).[4] In our opinion, it is most likely that the USPSTF criteria will be adopted when screening is implemented in the United States. In Europe and Asia the scenario may well be much more differentiated. In the United Kingdom, the current CT screening trial, the UK Lung Screening Study (UK LS), has more restrictive selection criteria, targeting individuals with greater than 5% lung cancer risk to increase cost effectiveness.[5–7] The remaining European screening trials have adopted enrollment criteria close to the NLST criteria, although most included individuals with 20 pack-year smoking history and age down to 50 years.[8–13] Screening compliance will also have a great influence on the number of persons that will actually be screened when CT screening programs are initiated. In the UK Lung Screen,[5,14] compliance was only 30%, and in the NLST only between 10% and 15 % satisfied the criteria.[15]

Screening Method and Lung Cancer Detection

In most trials including the NLST, screening has been performed annually,[2,10,11,13,16] but in the NELSON[17,18] and Multicentric Italian Lung Detection (MILD)[12] trials, both annual and biennial CT is evaluated. In the UK Lung Screen, a single CT screen approach has been adopted for the screening trial,[7] and biennial testing is evaluated before an eventual implementation of screening.[6] The USPSTF concluded that annual screening provides the greatest benefit in decreasing lung cancer mortality.[1,19] The NELSON trial has not yet reported their final results, but these are expected to have great influence on the policy in Europe. In the NLST, overall sensitivity of LDCT was 93.8% and was specificity 73.4%.[20]

The lung cancer detection rates depend on whether screening is a first (baseline) or subsequent incidence screening.[21] When discussing long-term effects of screening, it would seem most appropriate to use data from incidence screenings to simulate long-term implementation. One of the most critical issues raised by the NLST is the high false-positive rates of nearly 24%.[2] However, these rates may partly be explained by the lung nodule size cutoff criteria defining a positive screening result,[21] and only 2.5% of those with positive test results required further invasive diagnostic procedures.[2] In the European trials, false-positive and recall rates were much lower.[13,17,18] It is expected in the future that false-positive rates will be reduced by changes in definitions of a positive test result[22,23] and by extended use of radiologic volumetric software.[14,17,18,24]

In the NLST, a significant shift in lung cancer stages after screening was documented for the first time. This shift leads to an increase in frequency of lower lung cancer stages (stages I–II) and reduction in higher stages (stage III–IV).[2] Further analysis of the NLST data showed that the effect of screening on reducing in lung cancer mortality was dependent on the histology of the tumor. Patients with adenocarcinoma had the greatest reduction in mortality, and in squamous cell lung cancer, the effect was not significant.[25]

The number of lives saved by implementation of screening in the United States is estimated to be approximately 12.250 per year[15] and in the United Kingdom to be 956 lives saved per year.[6] The screening protocol suggested by USPSTF would result in a 14% reduction in lung cancer mortality or an estimated 521 lung cancer deaths prevented per 100,000 persons in the screened population. The harms associated with this screening protocol are an estimated overdiagnosis of 10% of screen-detected cases and radiation-induced lung cancer deaths of less than 1%.[1]

ONCOLOGIC IMPLICATIONS

A recent systematic review of lung cancer screening studies using LDCT found 8 randomized trials and 13 cohort studies.[26] The largest study by far is NLST in the United States,[2] which has given us the compelling data leading to implications for all specialties involved in lung cancer diagnosis and treatment. Below are some implications concerning the oncologic specialty outlined.

Implications of Changes in Disease Stage

In the NLST study, LDCT diagnosed more stage IA disease (416 cases of 1040 lung cancers detected [40.0%]) compared with CXR (196 stage IA of 929 lung cancers [21.1%]). There were no differences in stage IB through IIIA, but fewer patients in the LDCT group were in stages IIIB or IV (348 patients, 33.4%) than in the CXR group (457 patients, 49.2%).[2] The observed difference in stage IA would make no increased demand on oncologic resources, because this stage, with our current knowledge, does not require adjuvant chemotherapy after complete surgery, because no beneficial effect has been documented in this setting. Neither would there tend to be increased demand for radiotherapy for locally advanced disease because the frequencies of stages IIIA and IIIB were largely similar. However, the frequency of more advanced stages, such as stage IV and some stage IIIB, in patients who are candidates for medical antineoplastic treatment without curative intent, is lower for the group screened by LDCT. Also the need for palliative radiotherapy may theoretically be lower. This finding may suggest that LDCT screening may reduce oncologic treatment cost somewhat for the lung cancer field in general. It is, however, an open question to which extent these figures may be representative for the entire lung cancer population, because certainly not all patients have been included in screening programs but are diagnosed otherwise, even when a screening program is implemented.

Changes in Pathology

The NLST study is the only individual trial that has a reasonable power to detect possible impact in distribution of histologic subtypes discovered by LDCT screening. Most striking concerning histology in the NLST study is that the LDCT group comprised 110 patients having bronchioloalveolar carcinomas (10.5%) compared with only 35 patients (3.8%) in the CXR group.[2] Bronchiolaralveolar carcinoma is, with the current histologic classification, renamed to in situ, minimally invasive, or invasive adenocarcinoma with predominant lepidic growth.[27] This renaming may reflect the less-invasive nature of this histologic subtype, which also tends to be in lower stages. Hence, this observation seems not to impact on the demand for oncologic resources apart from the considerations mentioned previously.

Long-term Scenarios and Future Research Areas

If an LDCT screening program became fully implemented, and the question concerning the optimal population to screen takes into account benefit, harms, and costs, there will theoretically be a stage shift toward more disease being diagnosed, especially in stage IA, based on the NLST. Despite stage IA being the lowest stage of lung cancer, it is still a challenging prognosis, with a 5-year survival rate of 50% when clinically staged and 73% when surgically-pathologically staged.[28] Currently, no trials suggest that adjuvant chemotherapy will benefit these patients, even though a modest survival gain is shown when used in completely resected stages IIA to IIIA. Clearly, research on how to improve prognosis even in stage IA is important and will increasingly be so when more disease is diagnosed and patients undergo surgery in this stage. New drugs and biomarkers for new antineoplastic agents may be beneficial for individualized and, hence, improved adjuvant treatment.[29]

Knowledge is increasing on oncogenic driver mutations and their role in lung cancer development and treatment.[30,31] Among those with the currently drugable mutations, such as epidermal growth factor receptor mutation and anaplastic lymphoma kinase gen-rearrangement, most patients are somewhat younger have either no or low smoking consumption. Hence, these patients have another pathogenesis for their lung cancer and are accordingly not likely to be discovered by the current screening programs, as inclusion for these are based on somewhat older persons with a high tobacco exposition. The discovery by screening of lung cancers with relatively rare oncogenic driver mutations without the prevailing risk factors is currently not feasible. If at all feasible, it will take discovery of measures to enrich the screened population, but currently there are no tools for this.

FINANCIAL IMPLICATIONS
Costs of Computed Tomography Screening

The costs of implementing CT screening programs will inevitably vary greatly from country to country. International data may be transferable with regard to some epidemiologic parameters, such as etiology and risk, but clinical practices also vary between countries, and the costs of labor, equipment, and medicines are likely to be country or system specific. Each country will, therefore, have to make its own specific estimate, taking into account the specific character of the health care system, the defined screening-eligible populations, the screening participation rate, and the screening algorithm. The costs of the screening program additional to costs resulting from symptomatic presentation are (1) the costs of CT testing all individuals in the screening cohort, plus (2) costs of investigating all CT positives, plus (3) costs of treating the true positives, and minus (4) the costs of confirming and treating cancer among those who, in the absence of screening, would have presented symptomatically.[32]

Direct and indirect health care costs

The direct costs of the screening program are fairly straightforward to estimate. Indirect costs associated with CT screening may also be important but are more difficult to define and quantitate. The indirect costs include any costs initiated by the screening process. This may include increases in wages of screenees younger than retirement age (normally 65 years) who may live longer because of screening. In one evaluation, CT screening would actually lead to increased income and revenue leading to recovery of $0.38 of every dollar spent on screening.[33] In the DLCST (Danish Lung Cancer Screening Trial), it was documented that costs in the primary health care sector (general practitioner, physiotherapist, psychologist) were directly related to the results of CT screening,[34] and that a false-positive diagnosis led to increased health care costs also in primary health care. This study, for the first time, because of the randomized design and the Danish unique public registries, was able to show that CT-screened participants with a true-negative test result used the secondary and primary health care systems less than their counterparts in the control group who were not offered CT screening. As a consequence, the total cost of the screening program was reduced.[34]

Cost Effectiveness

After the demonstration of the mortality benefit in the NLST,[2] the cost-effectiveness analysis has been eagerly awaited but has not yet been published. Preliminary data suggest that it will be cost-effective with an Incremental Cost Effectiveness Ratio (ICER) of $72,900 US per quality-adjusted life year (QALY).[35,36] Previous estimates of cost effectiveness of CT screening for lung cancer have produced markedly different results.[32,33,37–41] In 2012, Goulart and colleagues[42] published a national analysis that predicted that LDCT screening would prevent 8000 lung cancer deaths in the United States. This was achieved at an additional cost of $240 per death avoided, based on the number needed to screen to prevent 1 lung cancer death. In a modeling study, McMahon and colleagues[40] concluded that the cost was between $ 126 and $169 per QALY gained. Villanti and colleagues[33] modeled the effect of annual CT screening for 15 years in a cohort of 18 million adults age 50 to 64 years with a 30 pack-year smoking history. The lung cancer screening intervention cost $27.8 billion over 15 years and gained 985,284 QALYs at an ICER of $28.24 per QALY gained.[33] They also found an additional benefit of adding smoking cessation intervention to the screening intervention, and calculated the cost at $23 per QALY gained.[33] The USPSTF did not include cost or cost-effectiveness estimates in their recommendation but did state that "current smokers should be informed of their continuing risk for lung cancer and offered cessation treatments. Screening with LDCT should be viewed as an adjunct to tobacco cessation interventions."[1] In the United Kingdom, the accepted incremental ICERs expressed as expected QALYs gained by screening was approximately £20.000 (approximately $37 US) per QALY in 2008, indicating that criteria for what is an acceptable ICER may differ between the United States and Europe.[32]

The calculation of the actual cost effectiveness of CT lung cancer screening will have to await the evaluation from the NLST and the final results from NELSON, DLCST, LUSI, ITALUNG, and other European trials. The indications from the NLST, however, are that CT screening may be cost effective.[35]

Long-term Scenarios

The effect of a screening program may be more pronounced in the long term when a screening program is fully implemented and has been running for years. The benefits may increase but the risk elements may also. With the rapid technologic development in diagnostic imaging that is expected within the next 10 to 20 years, it would be naïve to expect the screening technology to continue unchanged. On the contrary, changes and improvements are to be expected and anticipated. Resolution of CT images will no doubt increase, leading to earlier identification of suspicious lesions, but this may also increase the risk of false-positive findings even more than today. Surgeons may be asked to remove even smaller, 2- to 3-mm, nonpalpable lesions, which will require new technology developments. It is likely that imaging diagnostics in the future may make a preoperative tissue diagnosis unnecessary. The need for percutaneous or bronchoscopic markers of small nodules will no doubt increase to assist the surgeons.[43] It is unknown if the cumulative radiation exposure will be a problem or if it can be counteracted by future reductions in the CT screening radiation dose. The reading of CT scans by radiologist will no doubt be a great challenge because of the huge numbers of scans to be evaluated. Automated classification by computer aided detection (CAD) systems will be probably be developed, leading to fully automated analysis of CT screening scans, which may lead to a reduction in cost of CT screening.[24]

Current experience with screening trials has rarely exceeded 5 to 7 years.[13,16,18] In the DLCST, there was a decreasing participation rate after 4 annual years of screening[16] indicating that a fading compliance could be a long-term problem. It will be interesting to see to what degree the cost-reducing behavior of the large group of persons with true-negative CT screening results can influence the total costs of CT screening outside clinical trials. It seems probable that an increased focus on cost effectiveness, at least in Europe, will drive a demand for ways to reduce costs and increase benefits, such as the following:

1. Reducing the number of CT screenings by increased screening intervals[18]
2. Optimizing the risk profile of the screening cohort[6,14]
3. Development of more intelligent screening design based on findings of the first screening to predict the individual risk profile and creation of an individually tailored screening program[44]
4. Increased use of CAD systems may reduce costs of radiologist[24]
5. Combining CT screening for lung cancer with screening other diseases such as cardiovascular disease by coronary calcification scoring, emphysema and chronic obstructive pulmonary disease, and aortic valve stenosis.[24,45]

However, all of these will require further clinical trials to determine their efficiency and cost effectiveness.

SUMMARY

LDCT screening for lung cancer on a broader national scale will most likely be a reality within the next 5 years in the United States. In Europe, much will depend on the results from the NELSON trial and a pooling of results with other European trials. However, it will be a requirement that screening is cost effective and that the benefits of screening outweigh the drawbacks. The screening methodology will most likely continuously improve to achieve this aim and to provide hope for future generations of lung cancer patients.

REFERENCES

1. Moyer VA, U.S. Preventive Services Task Force. Screening for lung cancer: U.S. Preventive Services Task Force recommendation statement. Ann Intern Med 2014;160:330–8.
2. Aberle D, Adams A, Berg C, et al. Reduced lung-cancer mortality with low-dose computed tomographic screening. N Engl J Med 2011;365:395–409.
3. Jaklitsch MT, Jacobson FL, Austin JH, et al. The American Association for Thoracic Surgery guidelines for lung cancer screening using low-dose computed tomography scans for lung cancer survivors and other high-risk groups. J Thorac Cardiovasc Surg 2012;144:33–8.
4. National Comprehensive Cancer Network. National Comprehensive Cancer Network clinical practice guidelines in oncology: lung cancer screening. Fort Washington (PA): National Comprehensive Cancer Network; 2014.
5. McRonald FE, Yadegarfar G, Baldwin DR, et al. The UK Lung Screen (UKLS): Demographic profile of first 88,897 approaches provides recommendations for population screening. Cancer Prev Res (Phila) 2014;7(3):362–71.
6. Duffy SW, Field JK, Allgood PC, et al. Translation of research results to simple estimates of the likely effect of a lung cancer screening programme in the United Kingdom. Br J Cancer 2014;110:1834–40.
7. Baldwin D, Duffy S, Wald N, et al. UK Lung Screen (UKLS) nodule management protocol: modelling of a single screen randomised controlled trial of low-dose CT screening for lung cancer. Thorax 2011; 66:308–13.
8. van Iersel C, de Koning H, Draisma G, et al. Risk-based selection from the general population in a screening trial: selection criteria, recruitment and power for the Dutch-Belgian randomised lung cancer multi-slice CT screening trial (NELSON). Int J Cancer 2007;120:868–74.
9. Pedersen JH, Ashraf H, Dirksen A, et al. The Danish randomized lung cancer CT screening trial — overall design and results of the prevalence round. J Thorac Oncol 2009;4:608–14.
10. Lopes Pegna A, Picozzi G, Mascalchi M, et al. Design, recruitment and baseline results of the ITALUNG trial for lung cancer screening with low-dose CT. Lung Cancer 2009;64:34–40.
11. Becker N, Motsch E, Gross ML, et al. Randomized study on early detection of lung cancer with MSCT in Germany: study design and results of the first screening round. J Cancer Res Clin Oncol 2012; 138(9):1475–86.
12. Pastorino U, Rossi M, Rosato V, et al. Annual or biennial CT screening versus observation in heavy smokers: 5-year results of the MILD trial. Eur J Cancer Prev 2012;21:308–15.
13. Veronesi G, Maisonneuve P, Spaggiari L, et al. Diagnostic performance of low-dose computed tomography screening for lung cancer over five years. J Thorac Oncol 2014;9:935–9.

14. Field JF, Oudkerk M, Pedersen JH, et al. Prospects for population screening and diagnosis of lung cancer. Lancet 2013;382:732–41.

15. Ma J, Ward EM, Smith RA, et al. Annual number of lung cancer deaths potentially avertable by screening in the United States. Cancer 2013;119:1381–5.

16. Saghir Z, Dirksen A, Ashraf H, et al. CT screening for lung cancer brings forward early disease. The randomised Danish Lung Cancer Screening Trial: status after five annual screening rounds with low-dose CT. Thorax 2012;67:296–301.

17. van Klaveren RJ, Oudkerk M, Prokop M, et al. Management of lung nodules detected by volume CT scanning. N Engl J Med 2009;361:2221–9.

18. Horeweg N, van der Aalst CM, Thunnissen E, et al. Characteristics of lung cancers detected by Computer Tomography Screening in the Randomized NELSON Trial. Am J Respir Crit Care Med 2013; 187(8):848–54.

19. de Koning HJ, Meza R, Plevritis SK, et al. Benefits and harms of computed tomography lung cancer screening strategies: a comparative modeling study for the U.S. Preventive Services Task Force. Ann Intern Med 2014;160:311–20.

20. Church TR, Black WC, Aberle DR, et al, National Lung Screening Trial Research Team. Results of initial low-dose computed tomographic screening for lung cancer. N Engl J Med 2013;368:1980–91.

21. Seigneurin A, Field JK, Gachet A, et al. A systematic review of the characteristics associated with recall rates, detection rates and positive predictive values of computed tomography screening for lung cancer. Ann Oncol 2014;25:781–91.

22. Lam S, McWilliams A, Majo J, et al. Computed tomography screening for lung cancer: what is a positive screen? Ann Intern Med 2013;158:289–90.

23. Henschke CI, Yip R, Yankelevitz DF, et al. Definition of a positive test result in computed tomography screening for lung cancer: a cohort study. Ann Intern Med 2013;158:246–52.

24. Prokop M. Lung cancer screening: the radiologist's perspective. Semin Respir Crit Care Med 2014;35:91–8.

25. Pinsky PF, Church TR, Izmirlian G, et al. The National Lung Screening Trial: results stratified by demographics, smoking history and lung cancer histology. Cancer 2013;119:3976–83.

26. Bach PB, Mirkin JN, Oliver TK, et al. Benefits and harms of CT screening for lung cancer: a systematic review. JAMA 2012;307:2418–29.

27. Travis WD, Branbilla E, Noguchi M, et al. International association for the study of lung cancer/american thoracic society/european respiratory society international multidisciplinary classification of lung adenocarcinoma. J Thorac Oncol 2011;6:244–85.

28. Goldstraw P, Crowley J, Chansky K, et al. The IASLC Lung Cancer Staging Project: proposals for the revision of the TNM stage groupings in the forthcoming (seventh) edition of the TNM Classification of malignant tumours. J Thorac Oncol 2007;2(8):706–14.

29. Jakobsen JN, Sørensen JB. Intratumor variation of biomarker expression by immunohistochemistry in resectable non-small cell lung cancer. Eur J Cancer 2013;49:2492–503.

30. Siegelin MD, Borzuk AC. Epidermal growth factor receptor mutations in lung adenocarcinoma. Lab Invest 2013;94:129–37.

31. The Cancer Genome Atlas Research Network. Comprehensive molecular profiling of lung adenocarcinoma. Nature 2014;511:543–50.

32. Whynes DK. Could CT screening for lung cancer ever be cost effective in the United Kingdom? Cost Eff Resour Alloc 2008;6:5. http://dx.doi.org/10.1186/1478-7547-6-5.

33. Villanti AC, Jiang Y, Abrams DB, et al. A cost-utility analysis of lung cancer screening and the additional benefits of Incorporating Smoking cessation interventions. PLoS One 2013;8(8):e71379. http://dx.doi.org/10.1371/journal.pone.0071379.

34. Rasmussen JF, Siersma V, Pedersen JH, et al. Health care costs in the Danish randomized controlled lung cancer CT-screening trial: a registry study. Lung Cancer 2014;83(3):347–55.

35. Marshall HM, Bowman RV, Yang IA, et al. Screening for lung cancer with low-dose computed tomography: a review of current status. J Thorac Dis 2013; 5(S5):S524–39. http://dx.doi.org/10.3978/j.issn.2072-1439.2013.09.06.

36. Black WC. Cost Effectiveness of CT Screening in the National Lung Screening Trial, in 2nd Joint Meeting of the National Cancer Institute Board of Scientific Advisors & National Cancer Advisory Board 2013. Bethesda (MD). Available at: http://videocast.nih.gov/launch.asp?18018. Accessed August 19, 2013.

37. Mahadevia PJ, Fleisher LA, Frick KD, et al. Lung cancer screening with helical computed tomography in older adult smokers: a decision and cost-effectiveness analysis. JAMA 2003;289:313–22.

38. Wisnivesky JP, Mushlin AI, Sicherman N, et al. The cost effectiveness of low-dose CT screening for lung cancer: preliminary results of baseline screening. Chest 2003;124:614–62.

39. Manser R, Dalton A, Carter R, et al. Cost-effectiveness analysis of screening for lung cancer with low dose spiral CT (computed tomography) in the Australian setting. Lung Cancer 2005;48:171–85.

40. McMahon PM, Kong CY, Bouzan C, et al. Cost-effectiveness of computed tomography screening for lung cancer in the United States. J Thorac Oncol 2011;6:1841–8.

41. Pyenson BS, Sander MS, Jiang Y, et al. An actuarial analysis shows that offering lung cancer screening as an insurance benefit would save lives at relatively low cost. Health Aff (Millwood) 2012;31:770–9.

42. Goulart BH, Bensink ME, Mummy DG, et al. Lung cancer screening with low-dose computed tomography: costs, national expenditures, and cost-effectiveness. J Natl Compr Canc Netw 2012;10:267–75.

43. Field JF, Smth RA, Aberle DR, et al. International association for the Study of Lung Cancer Computed Tomography Screening Workshop 2011 report. J Thorac Oncol 2012;7:10–9.

44. Tammemägi MC, Katki HA, Hocking WG, et al. Selection criteria for lung-cancer screening. N Engl J Med 2013;368:728–36.

45. Rasmussen T, Køber L, Pedersen JH, et al. Relationship between chronic obstructive pulmonary disease and subclinical coronary artery disease in long-term smokers. Eur Heart J 2013. http://dx.doi.org/10.1093/ehjci/jet057.

Index

Note: Page numbers of article titles are in **boldface** type.

A

Agency for Healthcare Research and Quality
    and U.S. Preventive Services Task Force
        screening recommendations, 199–201
AHRQ. See *Agency for Healthcare Research and Quality.*

B

Biomarkers
    and populations eligible for screening, 218

C

Centers for Medicare & Medicaid Services
    and approval of low-dose computed tomography, 149–151
Chemoprevention
    and lung cancer screening, 161, 162
Chest radiography
    and cost of lung cancer screening, 205, 206, 210–212
    and Early Lung Cancer Screening Trial, 129, 130, 134–138, 140
    and lung cancer screening, 177, 178
    and Mayo Lung Project, 121–123
    and National Lung Cancer Screening Trial, 146–150
CMS. See *Centers for Medicare & Medicaid Services.*
Computed tomographic screening for lung cancer: The Mayo Clinic experience, **121–127**
Computed tomography screening: The International Early Lung Cancer Action Program experience, **129–143**
Continuous Observation of Smoking Subjects protocol
    and lung cancer screening, 162, 164, 166, 170, 171
COSMOS. See *Continuous Observation of Smoking Subjects protocol.*
Cost of lung cancer screening
    and annual health care expenditures, 209
    and areas for improvement, 209
    and chest radiography, 205, 206, 210–212
    and Early Lung Cancer Action Program, 206
    and health resource use, 209
    long-term implications of, 225–227
    and low-dose computed tomography, 205–215
    and National Lung Cancer Screening Trial, 205, 207–210, 214, 215
    and number of cases diagnosed, 211
    and review of literature, 206–208
    and U.S. Preventive Services Task Force recommendations, 205
Current estimate of costs of lung cancer screening in the United States, **205–215**
CXR. See *Chest radiography.*

D

Danish Lung Cancer Screening Trial
    and lung cancer screening, 162, 164, 178, 226, 227
DANTE study
    and lung cancer screening, 164, 167, 178
Detection rates
    and lung cancer screening, 224
Diagnostic algorithms
    and lung cancer screening, 161, 162, 164, 170, 172
Disease stage
    and lung cancer screening, 225
DLCST. See *Danish Lung Cancer Screening Trial.*

E

Early detection
    and lung cancer screening, 121, 168–170, 176
Early Lung Cancer Action Program
    background of, 129, 130
    comparison with National Lung Cancer Screening Trial, 135–139
    and cost of lung cancer screening, 206
    diagnostic mission of, 130, 131
    and lead-time bias, 133
    and length bias, 134
    and lung cancer screening, 129–140
    and overdiagnosis, 133, 134
    prognostic mission of, 131–133
Early Lung Cancer Screening Trial
    and chest radiography, 129, 130, 134–138, 140
ELCAP. See *Early Lung Cancer Action Program.*

F

False-positive results
    and lung cancer screening, 125, 126, 156, 157, 180, 181

Thorac Surg Clin 25 (2015) 231–234
http://dx.doi.org/10.1016/S1547-4127(15)00010-9
1547-4127/15/$ – see front matter © 2015 Elsevier Inc. All rights reserved.

Erratum

In the February 2015 issue (Volume 25, number 1), for the article "Candidacy for Lung Transplant and Lung Allocation," one author was listed incorrectly. The correct author name should be Carli J. Lehr, and the correct reference is Lehr CJ and Zaas DW. Candidacy for Lung Transplant and Lung Allocation. Thorac Surg Clin 2015;25(1):1–15.

Thorac Surg Clin 25 (2015) 235
http://dx.doi.org/10.1016/j.thorsurg.2014.12.007
1547-4127/15/$ – see front matter Published by Elsevier Inc.

Erratum

In the February 2015 issue (Volume 28, Number 4) in the article "Candidacy for Lung Transplantation: Lung Allocation," one author was listed incorrectly. The correct author name should be

Carli S. Lehr, and the correct reference is Lehr CJ and Zaas DW. Candidacy for Lung transplantation and Lung Allocation. Thorac Surg Clin. 2015;25(1):1-15.

http://dx.doi.org/10.1016/j.thorsurg.2016.12.007
1547-4127/15/$ – see front matter Published by Elsevier Inc.
thoracic.theclinics.com

Erratum

In the May 2014 issue (Volume 24, number 2), Awad A. El-Ashry, MD should be added as a co-author to the paper, "Total port approach for robotic lobectomy," by Robert J. Cerfolio, MD, MBA.

The new, complete reference should be: El-Ashry AA and Cerfolio RJ. Total port approach for robotic lobectomy. Thorac Surg Clin 2014;24(2): 151-6.

Thorac Surg Clin 25 (2015) 237
http://dx.doi.org/10.1016/j.thorsurg.2015.02.001

Printed and bound by CPI Group (UK) Ltd, Croydon, CR0 4YY

03/10/2024

01040377-0006